Physics MCQs for the Part 1 FRCR

Physics MCQs for the Part 1 FRCR

Shahzad Ilyas
Specialty Registrar in Clinical Radiology, Department of Radiology, Cambridge University Hospitals NHS Foundation Trust, Cambridge, UK

Tomasz Matys
Specialty Registrar in Clinical Radiology and Academic Clinical Fellow, Department of Radiology, Cambridge University Hospitals NHS Foundation Trust, Cambridge, UK

Nasim Sheikh-Bahaei
Specialty Registrar in Clinical Radiology, Department of Radiology, Cambridge University Hospitals NHS Foundation Trust, Cambridge, UK

Adam K. Yamamoto
Specialty Registrar in Clinical Radiology, Department of Radiology, Cambridge University Hospitals NHS Foundation Trust, Cambridge, UK

Martin J. Graves
Consultant Clinical Scientist, Department of Radiology, Cambridge University Hospitals NHS Foundation Trust, Cambridge, UK

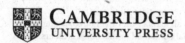
CAMBRIDGE
UNIVERSITY PRESS

CAMBRIDGE
UNIVERSITY PRESS

University Printing House, Cambridge CB2 8BS, United Kingdom

One Liberty Plaza, 20th Floor, New York, NY 10006, USA

477 Williamstown Road, Port Melbourne, VIC 3207, Australia

314-321, 3rd Floor, Plot 3, Splendor Forum, Jasola District Centre, New Delhi - 110025, India

103 Penang Road, #05-06/07, Visioncrest Commercial, Singapore 238467

Cambridge University Press is part of the University of Cambridge.

It furthers the University's mission by disseminating knowledge in the pursuit of
education, learning and research at the highest international levels of excellence.

www.cambridge.org
Information on this title: www.cambridge.org/9781107400993

© Cambridge University Press 2011

First published 2011

A catalogue record for this publication is available from the British Library

Library of Congress Cataloging in Publication data
Ilyas, Shahzad, author.
   Physics MCQs for the Part 1 FRCR / Shahzad Ilyas, Tomasz Matys,
Nasim Sheikh-Bahaei, Adam K. Yamamoto, Martin John Graves.
      p.   cm
   ISBN 978-1-107-40099-3 (pbk.)
   1. Radiology, Medical–Examinations–Study guides.   2. Radiology,
Medical–Examinations, questions, etc.   3. Radiologists–Examinations–
Great Britain.   4. Royal College of Radiologists (Great Britain)–
Examinations.   I. Title.
   R896.I49 2011
   616.07´57076–dc22

                                                        2010048121

ISBN 978-1-107-40099-3 Paperback

Contents

Preface

This book has been written by trainees who have successfully completed the new-style FRCR Part 1 physics exam and senior lecturers who have been chosen due to their renowned expertise in their specific field of work, providing the candidate with realistic exam-style questions, embedded with relevant facts and knowledge. The book is up to date in line with the new syllabus, with the inclusion of chapters covering MRI and ultrasound scans, and also covers new developments in legislation.

The questions in each chapter focus on the key concepts that are likely to be examined in that topic, allowing the candidate to test and reinforce their knowledge and identify areas of weakness. Clear and easy-to-understand explanations are provided with the relevant answers to allow the reader to understand the theory behind the questions.

The book has been written with the key focus of increasing knowledge of physics relevant to clinical radiology, making it an essential revision and learning tool for anyone sitting the new FRCR Part 1 physics exam.

Acknowledgements

We would like to thank the following for their help:

Dr Nicholas Bird MA MSc PhD MIPEM, Lead Clinical Scientist in PET/CT at Addenbrooke's Hospital, Cambridge, UK.

Stuart James Yates MSci, MSc, CSci, MIPEM, East Anglian Regional Radiation Protection Service, Cambridge, UK.

John Buscombe MD, FRCP, Consultant in Nuclear Medicine at Addenbrooke's Hospital, Cambridge, UK.

Mohamed Halim MRCP, MB ChB, Specialist Registrar in Nuclear Medicine at Addenbrooke's Hospital, Cambridge, UK.

and Richard Axell BEng(Hons), MSc, DipIPEM, Clinical Engineer, Addenbrooke's Hospital, Cambridge, UK.

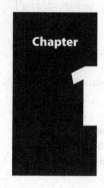

Chapter

1

Basic physics – Questions

S. Ilyas

1. Which of the following statements regarding protons are correct?
   a. They have a negative charge
   b. They are equal to the number of electrons in a non-ionized atom
   c. They are equal to the atomic number in a non-ionized atom
   d. They have no mass
   e. They increase in number relative to neutrons, following electron capture

2. The binding energy of electrons:
   a. Is the energy expended in moving an electron from an inner to an outer shell
   b. Is higher for an L-shell electron than an M-shell electron
   c. Is influenced by the number of neutrons within an atom
   d. Determines Bremsstrahlung photon energy
   e. Determines the energy of the photoelectron produced following photoelectric absorption

3. Which of the following are correct regarding electromagnetic radiation?
   a. Gamma rays are a form of electromagnetic radiation
   b. The particles have a mass equivalent to that of neutrons
   c. In a vacuum, the velocity of the particles differs depending on their individual properties
   d. It results in a sinusoidal graph when magnetic field strength is plotted against time
   e. The frequency is the interval between two successive crests

4. Regarding electromagnetic beam radiation:
   a. Energy fluence is the number of photons per unit area of a beam
   b. Beam intensity is the total amount of energy per unit area travelling per unit time
   c. Wavelength is inversely proportional to frequency
   d. Frequency is inversely proportional to photon energy (keV)
   e. Photon energy is inversely proportional to wavelength

5. Concerning electromagnetic rays:
   a. They travel parallel to each other in a straight line
   b. Beam intensity is proportional to the square of the amplitude
   c. The area of the beam is proportional to the square of the distance as it travels away from a point source

   d. Beam intensity is proportional to the square of the distance as it travels away from a point source

   e. The inverse square law is useful for estimating the intensity of a beam once it has passed through a copper filter

6. Which of the following statements are correct regarding an X-ray tube?
   a. The tube current (mA) is increased by increasing the filament voltage
   b. An increase in the tube voltage (kV) leads to a proportional increase in tube current (mA)
   c. Electrons are generated by heating the anode, which is usually made from tungsten
   d. The kinetic energy of electrons (keV) in the X-ray tube is dependent on the tube voltage (kV)
   e. The collision of electrons with a tungsten target mainly results in the production of X-ray radiation

7. Which of the following are true regarding the production of X-ray photons when using a tungsten target?
   a. The majority of X-rays emitted are a result of characteristic radiation
   b. The kinetic energy of electrons (keV) interacting with the target is equal to the kV between the anode and cathode of the X-ray tube
   c. Filament electrons with 90 keV can dislodge K-shell electrons in the target
   d. The energy of K_α radiation is greater than K_β radiation
   e. L-shell radiation makes up 25% of characteristic radiation emitted from the tube

8. Concerning characteristic radiation:
   a. It results in photons with a fixed energy, for a given material
   b. It mainly involves filament electrons dislodging L-shell electrons
   c. Photon energy is directly proportional to the tube voltage
   d. The rate of production of characteristic radiation is directly proportional to the filament voltage
   e. Atomic number influences photon energy of K-radiation

9. Concerning Bremsstrahlung radiation:
   a. It results mainly from filament electrons colliding with the nucleus
   b. It can result in photons that are equivalent in energy to the tube voltage
   c. It results in X-ray photons of the same energy, which are dependent on the target material
   d. An increase in atomic number of the target material results in an increase in the energy of photons
   e. A reduction in atomic number results in reduced photon production

10. Which of the following are true with regard to X-ray photon production?
   a. The area of a continuous spectrum graph represents the total output of all X-ray photons emitted as a result of characteristic radiation
   b. Increasing the tube voltage (kV) results in the continuous spectrum shifting to the right and the line spectrum increasing in height

   c. One-quarter of the photons from Bremsstrahlung radiation that reach the patient are less than 20 keV

   d. Increasing the filament voltage causes Bremsstrahlung and characteristic radiation graphs to increase in height

   e. Reducing the filament voltage has no effect on the maximum photon energy produced by characteristic or Bremsstrahlung radiation

11. Concerning the interaction of X-ray photons with matter:
   a. It is possible to predict the fraction of photons that will be absorbed or scattered, when passing through a given material
   b. Attenuation is represented by the number of photons absorbed or scattered by matter
   c. Scattered photons help form the primary image on the film
   d. The half-value layer (HVL) of a material is the thickness needed to reduce the number of photons in a beam by half
   e. The HVL is inversely proportional to the linear attenuation coefficient (LAC) of a material

12. Concerning factors affecting absorption and scatter of X-rays:
   a. An increase in the density of a material results in an increase in the linear attenuation coefficient (LAC)
   b. Increasing the atomic number of a material increases its half-value layer (HVL)
   c. Reducing the tube voltage increases the LAC
   d. Increasing the filament voltage reduces the HVL of a material
   e. A narrow beam has a higher scatter-to-transmission ratio than a wide beam

13. Concerning an X-ray beam:
   a. It reduces in equal quantities as it passes through material of equal thickness
   b. No matter how thick the material, it is not possible to completely absorb the primary X-ray beam
   c. Beam hardening results from a reduced number of photons being removed from the primary beam
   d. For a heterogeneous beam, the half-value layer (HVL) increases as the beam passes through the material
   e. Wearing lead gloves protects the operator's fingers from the X-ray beam

14. Which of the following are correct with regard to attenuation of X-ray photons?
   a. The Compton effect refers to the interaction of X-ray photons with free electrons
   b. Attenuation is the difference between the incident beam and the attenuated beam
   c. Photoelectric absorption refers to the interaction of X-ray photons with loosely bound electrons
   d. An increase in atomic number increases the linear attenuation coefficient (LAC)
   e. Elastic scatter results in no loss of energy

15. Concerning Compton interaction, which of the following are correct?
   a. It involves the collision of X-ray photons with any electron
   b. The probability that Compton attenuation will occur decreases as photon energy is increased
   c. Increasing the tube voltage results in a higher proportion of side scatter

    d. The higher the scatter angle, the greater the penetration of the recoil electrons

    e. An increase in the incident photon energy results in scatter photons with greater energy

16. Regarding the photoelectric effect:
    a. It results in the production of Bremsstrahlung radiation
    b. It results in the production of scattered photons, the energy of which is dependent on the initial photon energy (keV)
    c. X-rays passing through barium cause greater scatter than those passing through human tissues
    d. Ejection of a K-shell electron by an incident photon results in the production of an Auger electron
    e. Auger electrons are produced as an indirect result of photoelectric radiation

17. Concerning factors influencing attenuation:
    a. In material with a low atomic number, the photoelectric effect results in complete absorption
    b. The energy of the incident photon must be greater than the binding energy of the electron in photoelectric absorption
    c. An increase in the incident photon energy results in recoil electrons with lower penetration
    d. Reducing the tube voltage (kV) results in less scatter reaching the film
    e. The kinetic energy of the photoelectron ejected as a result of the photoelectric effect is not dependent on the atomic number of the material

18. Which of the following are true regarding the linear attenuation coefficient (LAC)?
    a. The photoelectric LAC is directly proportional to photon energy
    b. The total LAC is dependent on the physical density of the material
    c. The Compton LAC is dependent on atomic number
    d. The photoelectric LAC increases as the atomic number increases
    e. The Compton LAC is dependent on the electron density

19. Concerning absorption edges:
    a. K-edge binding energy is lower than L-edge binding energy
    b. Between the K-shell and L-shell, the increase in photoelectric attenuation is proportional to the photon energy
    c. For tungsten, the K-shell binding energy (Ek) is equal to 74 keV
    d. There is a sudden increase in attenuation when photon energy reaches L-shell binding energy (EL)
    e. When choosing a filter, it is important to make sure that the peak of the X-ray spectrum lies on the high-energy side of its absorption edge

20. Which of the following are true with regard to materials and attenuation?
    a. Following the Compton effect, the wavelength change of the X-ray photon depends on the atomic number of the material
    b. Photoelectric absorption is the predominating mode of interaction in modalities using high-energy photons

c. The Compton effect is the predominating mode of interaction in soft tissues
d. Photoelectric absorption is the predominating mode of interaction in air
e. The Compton effect is the predominating mode of interaction in contrast medium

21. Regarding secondary electrons:
    a. Positrons are negatively charged electrons that result from radioactive decay
    b. Beta particles can ionize atoms
    c. The collision of two positrons results in two gamma photons, each with 511 keV
    d. The range of the secondary electron is inversely proportional to the material density
    e. Secondary electrons result in biological damage of tissues

22. Which of the following are true with regard to filtration?
    a. The aim of filtration is to make the beam intensity more uniform by removing the very high-energy rays
    b. The tube housing acts as a valuable filter
    c. The predominant attenuation process in a filter should be photoelectric absorption
    d. At 80 kV, the half-value layer (HVL) of a beam with 2.5 mm Al filtration is typically measured as 2–3 mm Al
    e. The thickness of copper required to reduce the intensity of an X-ray beam by a factor of 2 is greater than the required thickness of aluminium needed to have the same effect

23. Concerning the effects of filtration:
    a. It increases the intensity of the beam
    b. It increases the half-value layer (HVL) of the beam
    c. It reduces the peak photon energy
    d. It reduces the effective photon energy
    e. It increases skin exit/entry dose ratio

24. Decreasing the tube voltage (kV) results in which of the following?
    a. It reduces the number of electrons colliding with the target
    b. It reduces the photon fluence
    c. It reduces the beam intensity
    d. It results in the increase of the half-value layer (HVL) for a given material
    e. The rate of photoelectric attenuation increases more than the rate of Compton attenuation

25. Which of the following increase X-ray beam intensity at a given point from a source?
    a. Increasing the filter thickness
    b. Increasing the tube current
    c. Increasing the distance
    d. Increasing the tube voltage
    e. Reducing the atomic number of the target material

26. Regarding the atom, which of the following are true?
    a. The mass number is equal to the number of nucleons
    b. Positrons are found within the nucleus

   c. The inner shell influences the chemical properties of an atom
   d. The outermost shell with electrons is known as the valence shell
   e. Radioactivity is dependent on the nucleus

27. Which of the following are correct with regard to X-ray production?
   a. Increasing the tube voltage increases the heat production at the target
   b. Reducing the actual focal spot reduces the heat load on the target
   c. Increasing the target angle increases the target heat rating for a given effective spot size
   d. Increasing the target angle increases the effective focal spot
   e. A rotating anode can take a higher heat load than a stationary anode

28. The nucleons in an atom:
   a. Reduce following beta-positive (β^+) decay
   b. Are equal to the atomic number
   c. Are equal to the difference between mass number and the number of protons
   d. May have a negative charge
   e. Affect the binding energy of electrons

29. Regarding photons:
   a. X-ray photons are produced following K-electron capture
   b. Collision of a positron with a negative beta particle results in the production of gamma photons
   c. X-ray photons are produced following photoelectric absorption
   d. They can be scattered only sideways or backwards following Compton attenuation
   e. They have a mass

30. Regarding radioactivity:
   a. Decay of radionuclides with a neutron excess produces a daughter nucleus with a higher atomic number
   b. The rate of decay can be increased by heating the radionuclide
   c. Isomers have the same half-life
   d. Decay of radionuclides with a neutron deficit produces a daughter nucleus with a lower atomic number
   e. Positron annihilation results in energy being converted to mass

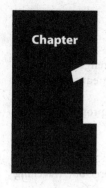

Basic physics – Answers

1. a. **False.** Protons have a positive charge. Electrons have a negative charge.
   b. **True.**
   c. **True.** Protons (atomic number (Z)) + neutrons ($A - Z$) = mass number (A)).
   d. **False.** Both protons and neutrons have a mass. Electrons have a negligible mass.
   e. **False.** Following electron capture the nucleus may increase its number of neutrons relative to protons by capturing an electron from the K-shell ($p + e \rightarrow n$)

2. a. **False.** Binding energy is the energy expended in completely removing the electron from the atom, against a positive force of the nucleus.
   b. **True.** The nucleus exerts a stronger pull on the inner electrons than the outer electrons.
   c. **False.** Neutrons have a charge of zero and hence do not affect the binding energy of electrons.
   d. **False.** Bremsstrahlung radiation is produced from filament electrons that penetrate the K-shell and approach the nucleus. Characteristic radiation is formed when an electron shifts from an outer to an inner shell, releasing a photon with energy equal to the difference in the binding energy of the two shells.
   e. **True.** In photoelectric absorption, when a photon collides with an electron from an inner shell, it ejects the electron, which is then termed a photoelectron.
   Kinetic energy of photoelectron (E_k for K-shell) = photon energy – binding energy.

3. a. **True.** Electromagnetic radiation is named according to how it is produced, e.g. X-rays (X-ray tube), gamma rays (radioactive nuclei).
   b. **False.** The different types of electromagnetic radiation differ in their properties and are made up of photons, which do not have a mass or electric charge.
   c. **False.** All forms of electromagnetic radiation travel with the velocity of light in a vacuum.
   d. **True.** Electromagnetic radiation produces a sinusoidal graph when electric or magnetic field strength is plotted against time or distance, travelling with velocity (C). The peak field strength is called the amplitude (A).
   e. **False.** Frequency (f) is the number of crests passing a point in a second. The interval between successive crests is called the period.

4. a. **False.** Photon fluence is the number of photons through a cross-section of the beam (i.e. per unit area). Adding the particle energies gives the total amount of energy per unit area and is called energy fluence.

b. **True.**
c. **True.** Wavelength is the distance between crests, when field strength is plotted against distance. Frequency multiplied by wavelength equals velocity ($\lambda \times f = V$)
d. **False.** Frequency is proportional to photon energy; the content of proportionality is called Planck's constant.
e. **True.**

5. a. **False.** Electromagnetic rays originate from a point source and diverge out, travelling in a straight line, unless attenuated.
   b. **True.**
   c. **True.** The inverse square law states that the intensity of radiation emitted from a point source will reduce in intensity, proportional to the square of the distance from that point, i.e. the area covered by the beam increases as the rays are diverging from a point; however, the number of photons remains the same and hence their intensity reduces.
   d. **False.**
   e. **False.** Important points to remember regarding the inverse square law are:
      i. Radiation comes from a point source.
      ii. There is no absorption or scatter of radiation between source and point of measurement.

6. a. **True.** The filament is heated by passing an electrical current through it, known as the tube current, which subsequently emits electrons.
   b. **False.** The tube voltage affects the kinetic energy of each electron (keV), not the tube current, i.e. number of electrons.
   c. **False.** Electrons are released by heating the cathode filament.
   d. **True.**
   e. **False.** The collision of electrons with tungsten results mainly in the production of heat, due to interaction with outer electrons.

7. a. **False.** Approximately 80% of X-rays emitted by a tube are Bremsstrahlung radiation.
   b. **True.**
   c. **True.** The kinetic energy of filament electrons needs to exceed the binding energy of K-shell electrons (70 keV for tungsten).
   d. **False.** For tungsten: K_α radiation = K-shell binding energy (70 keV) – L-shell binding energy (12 keV) = 58 keV. K_β radiation = K-shell binding energy (70 keV) – M-shell binding energy (2 keV) = 68 keV.
   e. **False.** As the binding energy of L-shell electrons is equal to 12 keV, the photon energy produced when an electron from an outer shell occupies the gap is too small to leave the tube (i.e. less than 10 keV).

8. a. **True.** Characteristic radiation results in the end production of photons that have the same energy, constituting a line spectrum, i.e. the difference in binding energies between the two shells, which is constant for a given material.
   b. **False.** It mainly involves filament electrons dislodging K-shell electrons.

  c. **False.** The tube voltage and filament voltage increase the rate of production of photons, but do not influence the photon energy, which is dependent on the atomic number of the target material.
  d. **True.**
  e. **True.** An increase in atomic number results in an increase in the binding energy of electrons and hence K-radiation.

9. a. **False.** Bremsstrahlung radiation mainly results from filament electrons penetrating the K-shell and being deflected by the nucleus, resulting in a loss of some of its energy in the form of a single photon.
   b. **True.** Rarely, an electron can collide with the nucleus, which completely stops it, resulting in a photon with the same energy as the applied tube voltage.
   c. **False.** This is true for characteristic radiation. However, Bremsstrahlung radiation produces photons with varying energies, resulting in a continuous spectrum.
   d. **False.** Increasing the atomic number of the target material results in an increase in the number of photons, but does not affect the photon energy, which is dependent on the energy of the electrons (keV).
   e. **True.**

10. a. **False.** The area of a continuous spectrum graph represents the total output of X-ray photons emitted as a result of Bremsstrahlung radiation, not characteristic radiation.
    b. **True.** Increasing the tube voltage increases the frequency of photon production as a result of characteristic radiation; however, it does not influence photon energy, which is dependent on the target material. Photons produced by Bremsstrahlung radiation increase in both their frequency and energy (keV).
    c. **False.** Photons with an energy of less than 20 keV are absorbed by the glass tube and do not reach the patient.
    d. **True.** Increasing the filament voltage increases the number of electrons colliding with the target material causing an increase in the number of photons produced by both characteristic and Bremsstrahlung radiation.
    e. **True.** Filament voltage does not influence photon energy in either characteristic or Bremsstrahlung radiation.

11. a. **False.** X-ray absorption and scatter are stochastic processes.
    b. **True.** Attenuation is the total number of photons that have been removed, as a result of scatter or absorption, from the primary beam after passing through the attenuated material.
    c. **False.** The X-rays transmitted through the patient form the primary image, while the scattered X-rays obscure it.
    d. **False.** The HVL is the thickness of a material that will reduce the intensity of a mono-energetic beam to half its value, not the number of photons.
    e. **True.** The LAC is the probability that a photon interacts (absorbed or scattered) per unit length it travels in a specific material. Hence, the greater the LAC, the lower the HVL of the material.

12. a. **True**. An increase in density results in a higher probability that a photon will interact with an electron as it passes through the material.
   b. **False**. An increase in atomic number results in a higher probability that a photon will interact with an electron (photoelectric effect) as it passes through the material and hence reduces the HVL.
   c. **True**. A reduction in tube voltage results in reduced photon energy, which means it is more likely to get attenuated as it passes through the material.
   d. **False**. Filament voltage increases the number of photons but not photon energy.
   e. **False**. A narrow beam results in a smaller amount of scatter.

13. a. **False**. This is only true for a mono-energetic beam. X-ray beams consist of photons with varying energies (poly-energetic).
   b. **True**. This is known as the exponential law.
   c. **False**. Beam hardening results from the low-energy photons being attenuated proportionally more than the high-energy photons as the beam travels through a material.
   d. **True**. As a result of beam hardening the penetrating power of the beam increases, resulting in an increase in the HVL.
   e. **False**. Protective equipment does not provide protection against the primary beam, only the attenuated rays.

14. a. **True**. The Compton effect is the interaction of X-ray photons with loosely bound or free electrons.
   b. **True**.
   c. **False**. Photoelectric absorption is the interaction of X-ray photons with an inner shell or 'bound' electron.
   d. **True**. An increase in atomic number results in a higher probability that a photon will interact with an electron (photoelectric effect) as it passes through the material.
   e. **True**. This also known as coherent scatter and occurs when the photon does not have enough energy to overcome the binding energy of an electron shell and hence 'bounces' off without the loss of energy.

15. a. **False**. Compton interaction refers to the interaction of incident photons with free or loosely bound electrons only.
   b. **True**. Attenuation generally decreases with increasing photon energies. However, the rate of decrease is much higher for photoelectric than for Compton attenuation.
   c. **False**. Increasing the tube voltage results in increased photon energy (keV) that in turn causes less side scatter.
   d. **True**. The greater the scatter angle, the greater the energy and range of the recoil electrons.
   e. **True**.

16. a. **False**. The photoelectric effect involves an incident photon removing a bound electron from its shell, resulting in the hole created being filled by electrons from outer shells, causing the emission of characteristic radiation.
   b. **False**. Unlike the Compton effect, the energy of the incident photon is completely absorbed after colliding with the electron and the photon disappears, resulting in no scatter photons.

c. **True.** Barium has a higher atomic number than human tissue and therefore produces characteristic radiation as a result of the photoelectric effect, with sufficient energy to exit the patient and act as scatter.

d. **False.** Ejection of the electron results in the production of characteristic radiation and an ejected electron (called a photoelectron).

e. **True.** The characteristic radiation produced as a result of the photoelectric effect is absorbed almost immediately in material with a low atomic number, resulting in the ejection of a further low-energy electron (Auger electron).

17. a. **True.** Characteristic radiation produced as a result of the photoelectric effect, in material with a low atomic number, has low photon energy and is absorbed almost immediately by the material.

b. **True.** Incident photon energy must be greater than the binding energy of the electron to eject it from its shell.

c. **False.** An increase in photon energy results in recoil electrons with higher energy and penetration.

d. **True.** Reducing the tube voltage causes a reduction in photon energy, having a two-fold effect:
   i.   There is more sideways scatter and less forward scatter towards the film
   ii. The scatter rays are less penetrating.

e. **False.** The energy of the incident photon, in the photoelectric effect, is taken up in removing the electron (binding energy) and the rest becomes the kinetic energy of that electron. Kinetic energy of photoelectron = photon energy – binding energy (Ek or EL). Hence, a higher atomic number results in a higher binding energy and therefore a photoelectron with a lower energy.

18. a. **False.** The probability that photoelectric absorption will occur decreases as the photon energy is reduced.

b. **True.** Total LAC = Compton LAC + photoelectric LAC. The density of the material influences both types of attenuation.

c. **False.** It is independent of the atomic number as it only involves interaction with free electrons.

d. **True.**

e. **True.** The probability that the Compton effect will occur is proportional to the physical density of the material, as well as to the electron density.

19. a. **False.** K-edge binding energy is higher than L-edge binding energy.

b. **False.** As photon energy increases, photoelectric attenuation decreases between the L-shell and the K-shell.

c. **False.** The atomic number of tungsten is 74. Its K-shell binding energy is 70 keV.

d. **True.** When photon energy reaches EL, interaction with L-shell electrons becomes possible and photoelectric absorption increases.

e. **True.**

20. a. **False.** The Compton effect is independent of the atomic number of the material as it only involves free electrons whose binding energy is negligible.
   b. **False.** As photon energy increases, the rate of photoelectric absorption decreases more than the Compton effect. Hence, at high photon energies, the Compton effect still predominates.
   c. **True.** The Compton effect predominates in low-atomic-number materials e.g. air, water and tissue.
   d. **False.** Photoelectric absorption predominates in high-atomic-number materials, e.g. lead and contrast medium.
   e. **False.**

21. a. **False.** Positrons are positively charged electrons that result from radioactive decay.
   b. **True.** Beta particles are produced as a result of radioactive decay. Similar to photoelectrons (photoelectric effect) and recoil electrons (Compton effect), they travel through material and interact with the outer shell of nearby atoms, resulting in them becoming ionized or excited.
   c. **False.** The collision of a positron with a negatively charged electron results in two gamma photons.
   d. **True.**
   e. **True.**

22. a. **False.** Filtration aims to remove a large proportion of lower energy photons, which are mainly absorbed by the patient and do not contribute to the image.
   b. **True.** The tube housing forms part of the inherent filtration along with the insulating oil, glass inserts and the target itself.
   c. **True.** Photoelectric absorption is inversely proportional to photon energy and therefore attenuates the lower energy photons.
   d. **True.** Total filtration = inherent filtration + added filtration.
   e. **False.** Copper has a higher atomic number than aluminium and hence a greater photoelectric absorption efficiency.

23. a. **False.** Intensity refers to the total energy per unit area, passing per unit time, which is reduced by filtration.
   b. **True.** Filtration results in beam hardening, resulting in a more penetrative beam, and causing an increase in HVL.
   c. **False.** Filtration causes the peak photon energy to increase, i.e. the energy level that the largest numbers of photons have.
   d. **False.** Filtration increases the minimum and effective photons, i.e. those that contribute to the image.
   e. **True.** Filtration reduces the skin dose while having little effect on the image.

24. a. **False.** The number of electrons (tube current, mA) is controlled by the filament voltage.
   b. **True.** Although the number of filament electrons produced are unaffected by kV, the number of photons created in the target per electron decreases with a reduction in kV, e.g. number of photos at 10 mA, 90 kV > number of photons at 10 mA, 60 kV.

   c. **True.** Beam intensity is the total amount of energy per unit area passing through per unit time.

   d. **False.** HVL reduces as beam penetration reduces.

   e. **True.** Due to a reduction in photon energy, the rate of photoelectric attenuation increases more than the rate of Compton attenuation.

25. a. **False.** This results in more photoelectric absorption of the low-energy photons and therefore a reduction in the total energy per unit area passing through per unit time (beam intensity).

   b. **True.** Increasing the tube current results in increased numbers of electrons colliding with the target and therefore increasing the number of photons produced by both characteristic and Bremsstrahlung radiation.

   c. **False.** According to the inverse square law, beam intensity is inversely proportional to distance, as long as the radiation is from a point source and there is no absorption or scatter.

   d. **True.** Increasing the tube voltage results in an increase in the kinetic energy of electrons colliding with the target, resulting in an increase in photon beam intensity.

   e. **False.**

26. a. **True.** Nucleon is a collective term for neutrons and protons. Mass number is the number of neutrons and protons in an atom.

   b. **False.** A positron is a positively charged electron that is ejected following radioactive decay.

   c. **False.** The outer shell (valence shell) influences the chemical, thermal and optical properties of an atom.

   d. **True.**

   e. **True.**

27. a. **True.** Increasing the tube voltage increases the kinetic energy of the electrons, the majority of which is lost as heat on collision with the target.

   b. **False.** This results in the heat being spread over a reduced area.

   c. **False.** The target angle is the angle between the target and the central photon beam. Reducing the target angle for a given spot size increases the area that the heat is spread over and therefore improves its heat rating.

   d. **True.**

   e. **True.** A rotating anode results in the heat being spread over a larger area and is one of the methods used to reduce target heating.

28. a. **False.** Nucleon is a term used to describe protons and neutrons. Beta-positive decay results in the conversion of a proton to a neutron plus an electron. Hence, the number of nucleons is unchanged.

   b. **False.** The nucleons equal the atomic mass (i.e. protons + neutrons).

   c. **False.** The difference between mass number and the number of protons is equal to the number of neutrons.

   d. **False.** Protons have a positive charge and neutrons have no charge.

   e. **True.** The number of protons (i.e. atomic number) influences the binding energy.

29. a. **True.** Characteristic X-ray radiation is released when an electron from the outer shell fills the hole in the K-shell left by the captured electron.
   b. **True.** Positrons collide with a negative beta particle resulting in the production of gamma photons with 511 keV each.
   c. **True.**
   d. **False.** Photons may be scattered in any direction; however, electrons are projected sideways or forwards only.
   e. **False.**

30. a. **True.** This is known as beta-negative (β^-) decay and results in the conversion of a neutron to a proton, therefore increasing atomic number.
   b. **False.** The rate of decay is dependent on the characteristic of the radionuclide and is unaffected by factors such as heat or chemical reactions.
   c. **False.** Isomers have differing half-life and energy states, but the same atomic and mass numbers.
   d. **True.** This can occur either by beta-positive (β^+) decay or K-electron capture, both of which result in the reduction of the number of protons and therefore atomic number.
   e. **False.** Positrons collide with negative beta particles resulting in the two masses being converted to energy.

Radiation hazards and protection – Questions

S. Ilyas and N. Sheikh-Bahaei

1. Concerning radiation damage to tissues, which of the following are correct?
   a. It is caused directly by photoelectrons
   b. Cells with high mitotic rates are less affected
   c. It is caused by free radicals
   d. Secondary electrons cause damage to tissue in a linear pattern
   e. It is caused directly by X-rays

2. Which of the following are true regarding dosimetry?
   a. Kerma takes into account the type of tissue being irradiated
   b. The absorbed dose is measured in grays (Gy)
   c. The equivalent dose takes into account the radiation weighting factor (w_R)
   d. The effective dose is measured in Gy
   e. $1\,\mathrm{Gy} = 1\,\mathrm{J\,g^{-1}}$

3. Regarding radiation dose:
   a. Linear energy transfer (LET) is the total energy deposited by a particle along its entire path
   b. An alpha particle has a lower LET than an electron
   c. Particles with high LET are more hazardous than low-LET particles
   d. The effective dose takes into account the radiosensitivity of the tissues
   e. $1\,\mathrm{Sv} = 1\,\mathrm{J\,kg^{-1}}$

4. Which of the following are correct regarding deterministic effects of radiation?
   a. It has a minimum threshold below which it does not occur
   b. The severity of the effect increases with dose
   c. The probability of the effect occurring increases with dose
   d. Breast cancer is a type of deterministic effect
   e. Skin erythema is a type of deterministic effect

5. Which of the following are correct regarding the stochastic effects of radiation?
   a. They can be hereditary in nature
   b. They arise as a result of chance
   c. The probability of the effect occurring increases with dose
   d. Increasing the dose results in an increase in the severity of the disease
   e. There is no threshold dose for stochastic effects

6. Which of the following are types of stochastic effects?
   a. Skin erythema
   b. Infertility
   c. Breast cancer
   d. Cataracts
   e. Leukaemia

7. Which of the following are correct regarding the principles of radiation protection?
   a. The dose to the patient should not exceed a certain limit
   b. Dose limits apply to workers
   c. The Ionising Radiation Regulations 1999 (IRR99) is concerned with radiation protection of patients
   d. The Ionising Radiation (Medical Exposure) Regulations 2000 (IRMER) is enforced by the Care Quality Commission
   e. The IRR99 is enforced by the Health and Safety Executive (HSE)

8. According to the Ionising Radiation Regulations 1999 (IRR99), which of the following are the responsibility of the employer?
   a. The employer should consult a radiation protection advisor on compliance with the regulations
   b. The employer is responsible for designation of the controlled area
   c. The employer is responsible for quality assurance of the procedures and protocols
   d. The employer is required to employ a medical physics expert (MPE)
   e. The employer should notify the appropriate authority if the dose to the patient is much greater than intended because of equipment fault

9. Local rules might include:
   a. Identification of who is permitted to operate the equipment
   b. Identification of who can refer a patient for X-ray
   c. Identification of those who may remain in the controlled area
   d. Setting the dose limit for controlled and supervised areas
   e. Notifying the authority if the wrong patient is radiated

10. Regarding workers and dose limits:
    a. The dose limit for carers is the same as for the public
    b. Trainees under the age of 18 must not receive an effective dose of more than 6 Sv
    c. Workers must be designated as classified if their annual dose limit exceeds 20 mSv
    d. Classified workers must be over 18 years of age
    e. It is mandatory to monitor the dose of all staff members who work with radiation

11. Which of the following could be radiation protection supervisor (RPS) duties?
    a. Overall responsibility for radiation protection
    b. Investigation of instances of excessive dose
    c. Ensuring staff follow the local rules
    d. Ensuring that an effective quality assurance programme is in place
    e. Risk assessment, e.g. for pregnant staff

12. Which of the following have been addressed in Ionising Radiation (Medical Exposure) Regulations 2000 (IRMER)?
    a. Regulation of medico-legal exposures
    b. Establishment of diagnostic reference levels (DRLs)
    c. Clinical evaluation of the outcome of every exposure and recording the dose
    d. Monitoring the classified person's dose
    e. Setting a dose limit for pregnant staff

13. An X-ray set fails to terminate properly during a chest X-ray examination because of automatic exposure control (AEC) failure. However, the back-up timer works and an investigation revealed that the patient received an unintended dose of ten times that intended. Which of the following statements are correct?
    a. It is necessary to inform the Health and Safety Executive (HSE)
    b. It is necessary to inform the Healthcare Commission
    c. The patient must not be informed of the incident
    d. A record of the investigation must be kept for 50 years
    e. The equipment should not be put back into use until the service engineer checks the equipment

14. It is a legal requirement:
    a. To report incidences when the wrong patient is given a medical exposure
    b. To carry out quality assurance measurements on diagnostic X-ray equipment
    c. To carry out representative patient dosimetry measurements
    d. To stop working with ionizing radiation if you have received a dose over the dose limit
    e. For employees to report suspected incidents involving radiation

15. Which of the following statements are correct regarding a patient's dose and the dose–area product (DAP)?
    a. The DAP can easily be measured and is directly related to the radiation risk
    b. The DAP can be converted to the absorbed dose using a conversion factor
    c. The conversion factors depend only on the region of the body, not the kV or filtration
    d. For the same region of the body, the conversion factor is the same for anterior–posterior (AP) and posterior–anterior (PA) views
    e. The entrance surface dose in the lateral spine view is more than that of the AP view

16. Regarding dose and hazards from X-rays:
    a. The dose from radiation scattered from the patient reduces roughly in proportion to the reduction in the area of the irradiated field
    b. A 0.25 mm lead apron will attenuate the scatter radiation by a factor of about 100
    c. Doubling the area of the X-ray beam approximately doubles the skin dose rate
    d. The effective dose to the patient can be measured directly using a thermoluminescent dosimeter (TLD)
    e. Someone in the primary beam at 2 m from the X-ray set could receive the effective dose limit in a few seconds

17. With regard to diagnostic reference levels (DRLs), which of the following are true?
    a. They are defined as the maximum dose for a particular examination
    b. They are adjusted according to the patient's body habitus
    c. They are set at the local level by the employer
    d. They can be assessed in terms of screening time
    e. If the DRL is exceeded, this must be reported to the Healthcare Commission

18. Which of the following are true regarding film badges in personal dosimetry?
    a. The film is highly energy dependent because of the intensifier
    b. The film has two different emulsions on each side
    c. The film can detect beta radiation and radioactive splash
    d. The aluminium filter will stop beta particles and the cadmium filter stops alpha particles
    e. As the film provides a permanent record of exposure, it can be used for more than 6 months

19. Which of the following are correct regarding thermoluminescent dosimeters (TLDs)?
    a. A TLD is not susceptible to environmental effects, especially high temperature
    b. A TLD shows a linear response to illumination and can be read only once
    c. TLD sensitivity is not significantly better than film
    d. A TLD needs a filter
    e. They can give readings down to 0.01 mSv

20. Which of the following are correct regarding electronic dosimeters?
    a. They are not highly energy dependent
    b. Their sensitivity can be 100 times that of a film badge
    c. They can be gas-filled tubes
    d. They do not need a filter
    e. They are useful in identifying methods of dose reduction for procedures with a potential high dose to staff

21. The approximate protection requirements for the walls/screens of a typical diagnostic X-ray room would be:
    a. 2 mm of lead
    b. 2 cm of glass
    c. 2 cm of barium plaster
    d. 2 cm of concrete
    e. 24 cm of brick

22. Regarding dose limits:
    a. The annual dose limit to the abdomen of women of reproductive capacity is 13 mSv
    b. The dose limit for the abdomen over the period of pregnancy for a pregnant employee working with diagnostic X-rays is 1 mSv
    c. The annual dose limit for the forearm in employees is ten times more than in members of the public
    d. The annual dose limit for a trainee is 6 mSv
    e. The dose limit for the lens of the eye for an employee at the age of 17 is 50 mSv year^{-1}

23. In terms of classification of staff and designated areas, which of the following are true?
    a. If an employee works in a supervised area, his external dose rate could be between 2.5 and 7.5 $\mu Sv\ h^{-1}$ averaged over the working day
    b. If an employee works in a controlled area it means that the dose to the lens of his eyes could be more than 45 mSv
    c. In a supervised area, it is likely that any person could exceed the dose limit for a member of the public
    d. Of the staff in the radiology department, 99% do not exceed the dose limit of a member of the public in any year
    e. If the finger monitoring of a radiologist showed that he received 150 mSv over the period of a month, it means he needs monthly dose monitoring and an annual health check

24. Regarding justification and optimization:
    a. Both referrer and practitioner must be registered medical professionals
    b. Both referrer and practitioner must have adequate training in radiation hazards
    c. The authorization is only given by the practitioner
    d. It is the responsibility of only the referrer and operator to make an enquiry about pregnancy
    e. Dentists, cardiologists and radiographers can act as referrer, practitioner and operator

25. A female worker who is operating an X-ray set when pregnant:
    a. Is advised to inform her employer in writing that she is pregnant
    b. Should report her pregnancy to the Health and Safety Executive
    c. Has a significantly increased risk of having a child with a genetic abnormality if she continues operating the X-ray set
    d. Will almost certainly have to alter her working practice
    e. Should desist from operating an X-ray set for the duration of the pregnancy

26. According to the recommendations for standard X-ray equipment:
    a. Leakage of radiation from the tube should be less than 0.1 mGy in 1 h at a distance of 1 m
    b. The total filtration in a dental setting should not be less than 1.5 mm of Al
    c. The collimator should be capable of restricting the field size to 10 cm × 10 cm
    d. The lead apron should not be less than 45 cm wide and 40 cm long
    e. For mobile equipment, the operator can stand at least 1 m from the tube

27. Which of the following statements are correct with regard to typical doses for radiological examination?
    a. A technetium-99m (^{99m}Tc) lung perfusion study results in the same dose to the patient as a technetium-99m bone scan
    b. Lumbar spine radiographs result in a higher dose to the patient than chest radiographs
    c. A barium enema typically results in a dose of 7 mSv
    d. A patient dose audit is part of the equipment quality assurance programme
    e. A computed tomography (CT) scan of the abdomen and pelvis results in a typical dose of 5 mSv

28. Regarding radioactive substances, which of the following are correct?
    a. The Environment Permitting Regulations 2010 are concerned with protection of hospital workers
    b. Medicines (Administration of Radioactive Substances) Regulations 1978 are concerned with the protection of patients from radioactive substances
    c. The Health and Safety Commission (HSC) is the governing body that issues the certificate for administration of radioactive substances
    d. Emptying the bladder reduces the dose to the gonads and pelvis
    e. The Administration of Radioactive Substances Advisory Committee (ARSAC) produces diagnostic reference levels (DRLs) or dose limits that should not normally be exceeded

29. In nuclear medicine:
    a. Radiopharmaceuticals with a shorter half-life result in a lower patient dose
    b. When preparing radiopharmaceuticals, syringes with a heavy metal sleeve block almost all radiation to the fingers
    c. Breast-feeding should be avoided for 72 h following administration of a radionuclide
    d. An ARSAC certificate is valid for 5 years
    e. The dose to the patient is directly proportional to the number of images taken

30. With regard to radiation protection of staff:
    a. The main radiation dose to staff in the room is from leakage radiation from the X-ray tube
    b. Standing close to the patient avoids scatter within the room and hence reduces the radiation dose
    c. Wearing lead aprons protects against the primary beam
    d. Under the Ionising Radiation (Medical Exposure) Regulations 2000 (IRMER), the equivalent dose to the lens of a classified worker should not exceed 150 mSv per annum
    e. Lead goggles can protect against cataracts

Radiation hazards and protection – Answers

1. a. **True.** When secondary electrons (e.g. photoelectrons and recoil electrons) pass through tissue, they result in ionization and excitation of atoms resulting in tissue damage.
    b. **False.** Cells with higher mitotic levels are more prone to radiation damage.
    c. **True.** Ionization by secondary electrons, results in damage to biological tissue either by rupturing covalent bonds or by the production of free radicals, which result in oxidation of organic molecules.
    d. **False.** Secondary electrons have a tortuous path, as negative electrons easily deflect them, leaving a track of ionized atoms behind.
    e. **False.** X-rays and gamma rays result in ionization of atoms via secondary electrons and are therefore indirectly ionizing agents.

2. a. **False.** Kerma is the kinetic energy of the secondary electrons released per unit mass of the irradiated material. It does not factor in the type of material being irradiated.
    b. **True.**
    c. **True.** Equivalent dose = absorbed dose × radiation weighting factor (w_R). It takes into account the absorbed dose and the type of radiation, e.g. X-ray, gamma ray or beta particle.
    d. **False.** The effective dose is measured in sieverts (Sv)
    e. **False.** $1 \text{ Gy} = 1 \text{ J kg}^{-1}$

3. a. **False.** LET is the sum of the energy deposited in tissue per unit path length it travels.
    b. **False.** Alpha particles are much heavier than electrons and hence for the same initial energy as an electron, they travel a much shorter distance and therefore disperse more energy per unit area travelled.
    c. **True.** High-LET particles disperse more energy per unit area travelled, resulting in more non-repairable damage.
    d. **True.** The effective dose incorporates factors to account for the variable radiosensitivity of organs and tissues.
    e. **True.**

4. a. **True.** Deterministic effect is characterized as having a threshold dose below which the effect will not occur.
    b. **True.** Once the threshold has been exceeded, increasing the dose results in the severity of the disease increasing.

   c. **False**. The effect occurs once the threshold is exceeded.
   d. **False**. This is a type of stochastic effect.
   e. **True**.

5. a. **True**. They may occur in descendants of individuals exposed as a result of lesions in the germinal cells.
   b. **True**.
   c. **True**.
   d. **False**. This is true of deterministic effects. Stochastic effects either occur or do not occur. Their severity is not affected by the dose.
   e. **True**.

6. a. **False**. This is a deterministic effect.
   b. **False**. This is a deterministic effect.
   c. **True**.
   d. **False**. This is a deterministic effect.
   e. **True**.

7. a. **False**. The dose to the patient should be as low as reasonably achievable (ALARA principle) in order to make sure that the patient receives maximum benefit with minimum risk.
   b. **True**. Dose limits apply to workers, such that a dose in excess of these values is deemed not to be justified, no matter how great the benefit.
   c. **False**. The IRR99 is not concerned with radiation protection of patients. Patient protection was introduced into UK law in the Ionising Radiation (Medical Exposure) Regulations 2000 (IRMER)
   d. **True**.
   e. **True**.

8. a. **True**. IRR99 Regulation 13: every employer must consult a Radiation Protection Adviser on compliance with the regulations.
   b. **True**. IRR99 Regulation 17: the employer should provide the local rules describing the controlled area and the working practice for these areas.
   c. **False**. Quality assurance of radiation equipment is a requirement of the IRR99, not procedures and protocols. The quality assurance requirements of the Ionising Radiation (Medical Exposure) Regulations 2000 (IRMER) are concerned with procedures and protocols and periodic audit of compliance.
   d. **False**. To have expert advice and ensure that an MPE is involved with medical exposure is a part of the IRMER.
   e. **True**. Incidents involving equipment faults are covered under the IRR99.

9. a. **True**.
   b. **False**. Identification of the referrer is a part of the IRMER
   c. **True**.
   d. **False**. Local rules include the description of controlled and supervised areas, not the dose limit.
   e. **False**. This is covered under the IRMER.

10. a. **False.** The IRR99 permits the dose limit to be relaxed for carers who are willingly exposed to doses higher than the limits set for the public.
 b. **False.** A non-classified worker (trainee) under the age of 18 should not receive a dose more than 6 mSv, not 6 Sv. Millisieverts (mSv) is commonly used to measure the effective dose in diagnostic medical procedures $(1 \text{ mSv} = 10^{-3} \text{ Sv})$.
 c. **False.** Workers are designated as classified if their annual dose limit exceeds 6 mSv. The effective dose limit for classified workers is 20 mSv.
 d. **True.** Classified workers must be over 18 years of age and certified as being medically fit, prior to employment, to work as a classified person.
 e. **False.** The IRR99 makes it mandatory to monitor the dose of classified workers only. In practice, the employer monitors the majority of staff working in a controlled area to monitor and keep dose limits within acceptable limits.

11. a. **False.** Overall responsibility for radiation protection rests with the employer.
 b. **True.**
 c. **True.**
 d. **True.**
 e. **True.**

12. a. **True.**
 b. **True.**
 c. **True.**
 d. **False.** This is covered under the IRR99.
 e. **False.** This is covered under the IRR99.

13. a. **False.** Regulation 23: if a patient has received a dose much greater than intended as a result of a defect or fault of the equipment, the HSE should be informed. A much greater than intended dose is defined as a multiplying factor of the intended dose in different types of examination. For chest X-ray, a dose of 20 times the intended dose is defined as much greater than intended.

Type of investigation	Multiplying factor
Interventional radiology, fluoroscopy, CT and nuclear medicine effective dose of >5 mSv	1.5
Mammography, nuclear medicine with effective dose of 0.5 mSv to <5 mSv, and anything else not listed in the table	10
X-ray of extremities, skull, dental or chest and nuclear medicine with an effective dose of <0.5 mSv	20

 b. **False.** If the overexposure is secondary to equipment failure, the HSE should be informed.
 c. **False.** The patient could be informed. However, when the dose is below the limit, it is not necessary to inform the patient.
 d. **False.** A record of assessment must be kept for 2 years.
 e. **True.**

14. a. **True.**
    b. **True.**
    c. **True.**
    d. **False.** Regulation 26: the employer must ensure that employees do not, during the remainder of the calendar year, receive a dose greater than the proportion of any dose limit that is equal to the fraction of the remaining dose limit period.
    e. **True.** Employees should inform either the radiation protection supervisor (RPS) or their employer regarding these incidents.

15. a. **False.** The DAP can easily be measured, but it is not directly related to the radiation risk.
    b. **False.** The DAP can be converted to the effective dose using the conversion factor.
    c. **False.** Conversion factors depend on the region of the body and to a lesser extent on kV and beam filtration.
    d. **False.** Conversion factors for PA examinations are less than AP examinations of the same region, because generally the organs and tissues with higher weighting factors are located anteriorly.
    e. **True.** The entrance surface dose in the lateral spine view could be around 10 mGy, while it is only around 4.3 mGy in the AP view.

16. a. **True.**
    b. **False.** A 0.25 mm apron transmits 5% of the scatter radiation.
    c. **False.** The skin dose rate will remain the same. However, the skin dose itself will increase.
    d. **False.**
    e. **True.** A few seconds is long enough for the primary X-ray beam to reach the dose limit.

17. a. **False.** DRLs are defined as doses for typical examinations of that type. They can be thought of as performance standards against which individual patient doses can be judged.
    b. **False.** They are set for standard-sized patients.
    c. **True.** They are set locally by performing patient dose audits.
    d. **True.** DRLs are set in terms of measurable quantities such as screening time, dose–area product and entrance surface dose.
    e. **False.** The patient dose may exceed the DRL for that examination, especially if the patient is overweight.

18. a. **False.** The film is highly energy dependent because of the high atomic number of silver and bromide. There is no intensifier in the film badge dosimeter.
    b. **True.**
    c. **True.**
    d. **True.**
    e. **False.** The film is subject to environmental effects such as heat, making it unsuitable for monitoring over long periods.

19. a. **False.** High temperatures can remove all the information from the TLD.
　 b. **True.**
　 c. **True.**
　 d. **True.** They are used in conjunction with filters set in the badge holder.
　 e. **False.** Optically simulated luminescent dosimeters can give readings down to 0.01 mSv. TLD sensitivity is similar to that of films (0.1 mSv).

20. a. **False.** Their response is highly energy dependent.
　 b. **True.** They are able to measure down to 1 μSv, while film sensitivity is not better than 0.1 mSv.
　 c. **True.** They can be based on Geiger-Müller tubes (gas-filled tubes).
　 d. **False.** They are placed behind a filter to give an accurate reading.
　 e. **True.** Because they provide a direct reading, they are useful for dose reduction for high-dose procedures.

21. a. **True.**
　 b. **False.**
　 c. **True.**
　 d. **False.** Generally, 150 mm solid concrete provides sufficient shielding.
　 e. **True.** 120 mm solid brick = 1 mm lead.

22. a. **False.** The dose limit in 3 consecutive months is 13 mSv.
　 b. **False.** The fetus dose limit is 1 mSv and it can be assumed that the fetal dose is no greater than 50% of the dose on the surface of the abdomen in diagnostic X-rays; thus, the dose limit for the abdomen could be around 2 mSv.
　 c. **True.** The dose limit for the hand, forearm, ankle and skin is 500 mSv for employees and 50 mSv for members of the public.
　 d. **True.** Dose limits for trainees are three-tenths that of general employees.
　 e. **True.**

23. a. **True.** In a supervised area, the dose rate is between 2.5 and 7.5 μSv h^{-1} averaged over the working day, while in a controlled area the dose rate could exceed 7.5 μSv h^{-1}.
　 b. **True.** The dose limit for the lens of the eyes is 150 mSv and a person working in a controlled area is likely to receive a radiation dose greater than three-tenths of any dose limit.
　 c. **True.**
　 d. **True.** Less than 1% of the staff in the radiology department whose dose is monitored receive more than 1 mSv in any year (dose limit for a member of the public).
　 e. **True.** A finger dose of more than 150 mSv per year means that the person should be classified. The monitoring period for classified workers is 1 month and they must have an annual health check and the records of these should be kept for 50 years.

24. a. **False.** Other healthcare professionals can act as a referrer.
　 b. **False.** Both practitioner and operator must have adequate training.
　 c. **False.** In special circumstances, the operator is given permission to authorize an examination.

    d. **False.** It is also the responsibility of the practitioner.

    e. **True.**

25. a. **True.**
    b. **False.**
    c. **False.**
    d. **False.** This is not true for the healthcare professional in a diagnostic setting.
    e. **False.** The dose limit during pregnancy is set such that it is equal to the limit for a member of the public, and for a diagnostic setting, it is highly unlikely to exceed this limit.

26. a. **False.** Leakage should be less than 1 mGy.
    b. **True.** In a general radiology setting, filtration should not be less than 2.5 mm of Al
    c. **False.** The collimator should be capable of restricting field size down to 5 cm × 5 cm.
    d. **True.**
    e. **False.** The operator should stand at least 2 m from the tube and X-ray source.

27. a. **False.**
    b. **True.**
    c. **True.**
    d. **True.** The Ionising Radiation Regulations 1999 (IRR99) require that patient dose assessment be part of the equipment quality assurance programme, making it important to audit patient dose.
    e. **False.**

Examination	Dose (mSv)
High dose (>2 mSv)	
CT abdomen or pelvis	10
CT chest	8
Barium enema	7
^{99m}Tc bone scan	4
Intravenous urography	2.5
CT head	2
Medium dose (0.02–2 mSv)	
Barium swallow	1.5
^{99m}Tc lung perfusion	1
Lumbar spine	0.8
Pelvis (AP)	0.6
Low dose (<0.02 mSv)	
Chest (PA)	0.015
Dental	0.004

28. a. **False.** The Environment Permitting Regulations 2010 are concerned with protection of the environment, with the enforcing body being the Environment Agency of England and Wales.
b. **True.**
c. **False.** The Administration of Radioactive Substance Advisory Committee (ARSAC) gives the certificate for administration of radioactive substances.
d. **True.**
e. **True.** In nuclear medicine, the dose is kept within the DRLs set by the ARSAC.

29. a. **True.** The dose to an organ increases in proportion to the following:
i. The effective half-life
ii. The fraction taken up by the organ
iii. The activity administered to the patient
iv. The energy of alpha and beta radiation emitted.
b. **False.**
c. **False.** Breast-feeding should be avoided for 24 h.
d. **True.**
e. **False.** The number of images taken is independent of the dose to the patient in nuclear medicine examination.

30. a. **False.** Leakage radiation from the X-ray tube is than 2% of the dose received by staff in the room. Scatter radiation from Compton interaction within the patient is the main radiation dose to staff.
b. **False.** The principles of radiation protection are:
i. Time: the shorter the exposure time, the lower the dose received
ii. Distance: the inverse square law states that the intensity of the beam reduces from a source as distance increases
iii. The thicker/denser the material, the better the shielding it provides.
c. **False.**
d. **False.** The Ionising Radiation Regulations 1999 (IRR99) are concerned with setting dose limits for worker, not the IRMER. The equivalent dose limit for the lens of a classified worker should not exceed 150 mSv per annum.
e. **True.** Lead goggles are often used by interventionists.

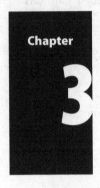

Imaging with X-rays – Questions

T. Matys and A. K. Yamamoto

1. Regarding subject contrast in radiography, which of the following are correct?
   a. It depends on the thickness of the structure being imaged
   b. It depends on the linear attenuation coefficients of the structures being imaged
   c. It increases with the tube kV
   d. Contrast between low-atomic-number structures (e.g. fat and muscle) is strongly affected by changes in the tube kV
   e. Contrast between air and soft tissue is due to differences in their atomic numbers

2. Concerning radiographic contrast:
   a. Attenuation of the X-ray beam depends upon the degree of Bremsstrahlung in the tissue
   b. Most structures on a chest radiograph exhibit good radiographic contrast
   c. In principle, contrast media have the same effect on demonstrating contrast between tissues as increasing the peak kV (kVp)
   d. All contrast media attenuate X-rays to a higher degree than the tissue
   e. Positive-contrast media should generally have high atomic numbers to maximize the degree of photoelectric absorption

3. Which of the following are correct for positive-contrast media?
   a. They should ideally have an absorption edge just to the left of the major part of the beam spectrum
   b. Barium has a K-absorption edge of approximately 23 keV
   c. Iodine has a lower atomic number than barium
   d. Iodine most effectively attenuates photons with energies close to 37 keV
   e. They may produce characteristic radiation

4. Concerning magnification:
   a. It occurs because X-rays converge on the object
   b. Assuming a fixed focal spot position, it increases as the object is moved nearer to the film
   c. Assuming a fixed position of the object in relation to the focal spot, it increases as the focus-to-film distance (FFD) is increased
   d. If the object is in contact with the film, the magnification factor is 1
   e. Minification of the image with film-screen radiography cannot occur

5. Geometric unsharpness:
   a. Occurs because X-ray photons are emitted from an area of finite size rather than from a point source

   b. Increases with focal spot size
   c. Decreases with shortening of the object-to-film distance
   d. Increases with shortening of the focus-to-film distance
   e. Decreases towards the anode side of the image

6. Regarding movement (motion) unsharpness:
   a. It can be reduced by immobilization
   b. It can be reduced by using a short exposure time
   c. It can be exaggerated by increasing the object-to-film distance
   d. Increasing the focus-to-film distance always decreases movement unsharpness
   e. Shortening the exposure time to overcome the motion unsharpness may contribute to increased geometric unsharpness

7. Concerning the focal spot:
   a. The area of the anode over which electrons are targeted is the actual focal spot
   b. The size of the effective focal spot is the same as the actual focal spot
   c. The anode angle is the angle between the central X-ray beam and the target face
   d. The value of the anode angle is usually in the range of 7–30°
   e. Increasing the anode angle increases the actual focal spot size

8. Concerning the focal spot:
   a. A larger actual focal spot allows greater tube currents
   b. Increasing the anode angle increases the maximum permissible exposure factors that can be used
   c. A typical size of focal spot in general radiography is 1 mm
   d. Focal spot size has no effect on contrast
   e. A larger focal spot size increases the amount of scatter

9. Concerning the focal spot:
   a. Its size may be estimated using a slit camera
   b. Its size may be estimated using a star test pattern
   c. A smaller anode angle reduces the size of the effective focal spot
   d. A larger anode angle is useful for general radiography
   e. The size of the actual focal spot is partly determined by the length of the cathode filament

10. The heel effect:
   a. Is due to attenuation of electrons in the target material
   b. Is greater on the cathode side of the X-ray field
   c. Is more pronounced at small anode angles
   d. Is more noticeable at high peak kV (kVp)
   e. Results in higher mean energy spectrum of the beam on the anode side compared to the cathode side

11. Regarding the heel effect:
   a. It is more pronounced in worn-out anodes with a rugged surface
   b. It is less pronounced in tubes with rotating compared with stationary anodes

c. For a given film size, it is more noticeable on images acquired with a long focus-to-film distance
d. In mammography, the anode side of the tube should be directed towards the chest wall
e. It is useful in spine radiographs

12. Regarding X-ray tube operation:
   a. Peak kV (kVp) and mA may be varied independently of one another
   b. For a given anode, the focal spot size cannot be varied
   c. Exposure settings may be set automatically by the system
   d. Automatic exposure control (AEC) is usually used
   e. mA and exposure time are usually adjusted simultaneously

13. Which of the following are true about the quality and quantity of the X-ray beam?
   a. The quality describes the number of photons in the X-ray beam
   b. The quantity determines the penetrability of the X-ray beam
   c. The quantity is inversely proportional to the tube current
   d. The quantity is directly proportional to the tube voltage
   e. The quantity is dependent on the choice of target material in the anode

14. Concerning exposure controls:
   a. Automatic exposure control (AEC) can be varied to adjust the optical density of the film
   b. A faulty AEC detector will usually result in significant overexposure of the patient
   c. AEC is more likely to ensure the correct exposure when used with collimation
   d. AEC typically uses five ionization chambers
   e. All ionization chambers must be used simultaneously

15. Regarding collimation:
   a. It allows the operator to adjust the filtration of the X-ray beam
   b. It employs a light beam diaphragm
   c. The collimators are constructed of material that is highly attenuating to X-rays
   d. It reduces scatter
   e. It does not affect the effective dose to the patient

16. Regarding the X-ray tube anode:
   a. It is the site of thermionic emission
   b. Tungsten is a suitable target material
   c. Electrons striking the anode mostly convert their energy into X-ray photons
   d. It is usually rotating
   e. The anode material used in mammography is the same as in general radiology

17. Regarding the construction of a rotating anode X-ray tube:
   a. The entire anode disc is usually made of tungsten
   b. The anode stem is made of molybdenum to improve the conduction of heat away from the anode disc
   c. The rotor bearings are lubricated with a soft metal

    d. The electric brushes of the X-ray tube motor are made of graphite

    e. The filament assembly is aligned with the anode stem

18. With regard to the cooling of a rotating anode X-ray tube:

    a. Heat produced in the focal spot is transferred to the glass envelope by convection

    b. Heat is transferred out of the tube housing into the atmosphere by conduction

    c. The anode assembly is blackened to improve radiation of heat

    d. The major thermal limiting factor for single exposures is the heat capacity of the focal spot area

    e. In the case of continuous/repeated exposures, the major limiting factor is the heat capacity of the anode disc and the tube housing

19. Regarding the high-voltage supply to the X-ray tube:

    a. In a self-rectified tube, X-rays are produced during both the positive and the negative halves of the supplying voltage waveform

    b. In a tube connected to a half-wave rectifying circuit, X-rays are produced during both halves of the supplying voltage waveform

    c. In a fully rectified one-phase circuit, the voltage across the tube is almost constant

    d. A fully rectified three-phase supply provides more constant voltage throughout the cycle than a one-phase supply

    e. A tube supplied from a high-frequency generator requires less filtration in comparison with that supplied from rectified circuits

20. Regarding factors affecting X-ray emission:

    a. The tube voltage affects the maximum energy of Bremsstrahlung radiation

    b. Due to inherent tube filtration, the maximum energy of photons measured in keV is slightly lower than the tube potential in kV

    c. Beam filtration affects both the quantity and quality of the X-ray beam

    d. Increasing peak kV (kVp) increases the quantity and quality of the emitted X-ray beam

    e. Increasing the tube current decreases the half-value layer (HVL) of the beam

21. X-ray exposure ratings:

    a. Determine the operational limits of the X-ray equipment

    b. May be illustrated graphically

    c. Are independent of focal spot size

    d. Are dependent on the anode rotation speed

    e. Are the same for single and repeated exposures

22. Regarding patient dose in radiography:

    a. The ratio of entrance surface dose (ESD) to exit dose is similar in most radiographic examinations

    b. The film dose required to produce an image in film-screen radiography is in the range of 0.2–0.5 µGy

    c. Increasing mAs increases the exit dose and ESD proportionately

    d. Increasing the tube kV increases the ratio of ESD to the exit dose

    e. Increasing filtration reduces the ratio of ESD to the exit dose

23. Patient dose in radiography can be reduced by:
    a. Increasing the focus-to-film distance
    b. Compression
    c. Collimation
    d. Using a secondary radiation grid
    e. Using the air-gap technique

24. The amount of scattered radiation leaving the patient is decreased by:
    a. Decreasing the tube kV
    b. Reducing the field area by collimation
    c. Compression of the patient
    d. Using a radiation grid
    e. Using the air-gap technique

25. Increasing the focus-to-film distance while keeping the film exposure constant:
    a. Improves radiographic contrast
    b. Reduces patient dose
    c. Reduces magnification
    d. Reduces geometric unsharpness
    e. Improves field uniformity

26. Regarding the construction of a radiation grid:
    a. It is made of 0.05–0.07 mm lead strips
    b. The line density of a grid is usually 12–16 cm^{-1}
    c. The gaps between the lead strips are filled with air
    d. The grid ratio is the ratio of the depth of the interspace channel divided by its width
    e. A typical grid ratio is 30:1–80:1

27. Concerning radiation grids:
    a. A parallel grid is focused at infinity
    b. For a focused grid, the focusing range depends on the grid ratio
    c. In the case of a crossed grid composed of two linear grids, the resulting grid ratio is equal to the product of individual grid ratios
    d. The contrast improvement factor of a typical grid is 2–4
    e. Grids are generally not used in paediatric radiography

28. Regarding dual-energy radiography:
    a. It exploits spectral differences in X-ray attenuation by various tissues
    b. It may be used to produce selective tissue images
    c. It always requires two separate exposures
    d. In dual-exposure systems for chest radiography, tube potentials of 60 and 120 kV are usually used
    e. Dual-exposure systems are prone to misregistration artefacts

29. Concerning dual-energy radiography:
    a. Dual-exposure systems produce selective tissue images with a better signal-to-noise ratio than single-exposure systems
    b. It requires slightly lower radiation doses than conventional radiography

   c. It is most commonly used in chest imaging
   d. It helps detect calcium within soft tissue structures
   e. Three images are typically produced for reporting

30. Regarding quality assurance in radiography:
   a. The tube kV is tested using a dosimeter
   b. Tube output is assessed with an ionization chamber or a solid-state detector
   c. For a given mAs, the output of the tube should be constant over the entire voltage range
   d. Tube filtration is assessed by measuring the half-value layer (HVL)
   e. Light beam diaphragm alignment should be checked yearly.

Chapter 3

Imaging with X-rays – Answers

1. a. **True**. It is proportional to the thickness of the imaged object.
   b. **True**. It is proportional to the difference between linear attenuation coefficients of the tissues involved.
   c. **False**. With increasing peak kV (kVp), the relative probability of the Compton effect increases, which compromises contrast.
   d. **False**. In the range of photon energies used in general radiography, the contrast between low-atomic-number tissues is low and only minimally dependent on kVp.
   e. **False**. It is due to a large difference in density. The effective atomic numbers of air and soft tissue are very similar.

2. a. **False**. Attenuation is due to Compton scattering and photoelectric absorption. Bremsstrahlung relates to the production of X-rays.
   b. **True**. This is due to the different attenuation properties of air, fat, soft tissue and bone (the main four 'radiographic densities').
   c. **False**. As they improve contrast, their effect is analogous to decreasing the peak kV (kVp).
   d. **False**. Negative-contrast media (for example, air or carbon dioxide) are radiolucent.
   e. **True**.

3. a. **True**.
   b. **False**. This is the value for rhodium. Barium has an absorption edge of 37 keV.
   c. **True**. The atomic numbers of iodine and barium are 53 and 56, respectively.
   d. **False**. As the K-absorption edge of iodine is 33 keV, it is most effective in attenuating photons of this energy. The answer to this question would be true for barium.
   e. **True**. This happens when an electron within the K-shell is ejected and replaced by an electron from another valence band.

4. a. **False**. It occurs because X-rays are divergent from their source.
   b. **False**. This decreases magnification.
   c. **True**. The object-to-film distance would increase.
   d. **True**. In this case, there would be no magnification.
   e. **True**.

5. a. **True**.
   b. **True**. The larger the focal spot size, the larger the penumbra (image blur around the edges of an object).
   c. **True**. The closer the object to the detector, the less unsharpness.

d. **True.** The closer the focus to the film, the more geometric unsharpness. In summary, geometric unsharpness depends on the focal spot size (f), object-to-film distance (h) and focus-to-film distance (FFD) and is given by the formula $U_g = fh/(FFD - h)$.

e. **True.** This is because the projected focal spot decreases in size towards the anode side.

6. a. **True.** However, this may not always be possible (e.g. in case of movement blur due to heart beating).

b. **True.**

c. **True.** In this case, the same amount of object movement will translate to a larger distance on the film.

d. **False.** It may increase motion blur as it necessitates increased exposure time.

e. **True.** This is because to expose the film in a shorter time, the tube current needs to be increased, which may require selecting a larger focal spot. The size of the focal spot may also increase with a higher tube current due to the blooming effect.

7. a. **True.**

b. **False.** The effective focal spot is the area of the actual focal spot viewed from the film. Due to anode angulation, it is smaller than the actual focal spot.

c. **True.**

d. **False.** It is usually 7–20°.

e. **True.**

8. a. **True.**

b. **True.** Increasing the anode angle increases the size of the actual focal spot and so a greater tube current or kVp may be used.

c. **True.**

d. **True.**

e. **False.** It does not affect scatter.

9. a. **True.** A slit camera consists of a metal plate with a slit positioned between the tube and the image receptor. One dimension of the focal spot can be calculated from magnification of the slit image. This is then repeated for the other dimension with the slit perpendicular to its original position.

b. **True.** This involves a test object with markings at a set distance apart with which an image is produced of a certain magnification. The degree of blurring of the markings in the image can be used to estimate focal spot size, as it is greater with a larger focal spot.

c. **True.**

d. **True.** This allows greater tube loading and higher output, which is often necessary when imaging larger parts of the body. It also increases the size of the field coverage at short focal spot-to-image distances.

e. **True.** It is also determined by the width of the focusing cup at the cathode.

10. a. **False.** It is due to attenuation of X-ray photons produced by the target material.

b. **False.** Due to anode angulation, photons emitted towards the anode side of the field need to penetrate a larger thickness of the anode material and therefore undergo more attenuation.

   c. **True**. The steeper the target, the larger the thickness of the target material that needs to be penetrated on the anode side.

   d. **False**. It is more noticeable at low kVp, as the photons are less penetrating and the differences in attenuation on the cathode and anode sides are more pronounced.

   e. **True**. Because photons penetrating through the target material in addition to attenuation also undergo filtration.

11. a. **True**. The electrons penetrate deeper into the anode material and the photons produced have a greater distance to travel through it.

   b. **False**. Anode rotation does not directly affect the heel effect. However, the heel effect is of less significance in stationary anodes tubes as they tend to have larger anode angles (due to thermal factors), and the field uniformity is not as critical in the applications they are used in.

   c. **False**. With a long focus-to-film distance, only the central, more uniform part of the beam is used to produce the image and the heel effect is less noticeable.

   d. **False**. The anode side (with a lower intensity of the beam due to the heel effect) should point away from the chest wall (where the thickness of breast tissue is less).

   e. **True**. It may be used to compensate for varying patient thickness along the cranio-caudal axis. For example, antero-posterior (AP) images of the thoracic spine are normally more penetrated (darker) towards the upper vertebrae. With the anode facing cranially, more uniform images can be obtained.

12. a. **True**.

   b. **False**. This may be achieved by choosing a different filament length (there are usually two). Some anode discs may also have bevels at different inclinations allowing the choice of a different anode angle.

   c. **True**. This may be achieved automatically by anatomically programmed radiography (APR), which will set the kVp/mA/exposure time depending on the particular projection.

   d. **True**. AEC uses a radiation detector (usually an ionization chamber) placed in close proximity to the image plate, terminating exposure when a sufficient quantity of radiation has reached the film. This is especially important in computed/digital radiography where the detector has a large latitude, and the choice of excessive parameters does not result in obvious overexposure.

   e. **True**. They are usually adjusted as a single parameter (mAs).

13. a. **False**. This is the quantity.

   b. **False**. X-ray beam penetrability is dependent on beam quality. An X-ray beam containing higher energy photons is more penetrating.

   c. **False**. It is directly proportional.

   d. **False**. In the range of tube voltages used in general radiography, it is approximately proportional to the square of peak kV (kVp).

   e. **True**. The amount of Bremsstrahlung radiation produced in higher-atomic-number targets is greater.

14. a. **True**. The operator can adjust the AEC to produce an image of a certain optical density, known as the density setting.
   b. **False**. This should be prevented by a back-up timer, which terminates the exposure if the AEC fails to do so, usually when 150% of expected manual exposure is reached.
   c. **True**.
   d. **False**. There are usually three chambers covering different areas of the film.
   e. **False**. The operator can select which chambers to use depending on the projection.

15. a. **False**. It allows adjustment of the beam size. It has no effect on filtration.
   b. **True**. This is a light source that projects as though it originated from the X-ray focus, allowing the operator to see the position of the beam projected onto the patient.
   c. **True**.
   d. **True**. Less tissue is irradiated by directing the X-ray beam onto a smaller target area.
   e. **False**. It decreases the volume of tissue irradiated and the radiation dose.

16. a. **False**. Thermionic emission occurs in the cathode, and the released electrons are targeted on the anode target.
   b. **True**. This is due to its high melting point and high atomic number ($Z = 74$), which increases the degree of Bremsstrahlung.
   c. **False**. The energy of the electrons is mainly converted into heat, which is why the anode must be able to tolerate a significant temperature rise. Less than 1% is converted to X-ray photons.
   d. **True**. The anode may be stationary or rotating. Rotating anodes are used for better tolerance of the heat generated during the production of X-rays, as the heat is spread over a larger area.
   e. **False**. Rhodium ($Z = 45$) and molybdenum ($Z = 42$) are chosen due to the useful energies of characteristic radiation.

17. a. **False**. It is usually made of molybdenum, in which the target annulus (made of tungsten alloy) is embedded.
   b. **False**. The opposite is true. Molybdenum has a low heat conductivity, which slows the conduction of heat towards the rotor bearings, protecting them from heat damage.
   c. **True**. They are usually lubricated with silver powder.
   d. **False**. Induction motors are used. These are brushless.
   e. **False**. The filament is offset towards the edge of the anode, in line with the target annulus.

18. a. **False**. It is conducted to the anode disc and transfers to the glass envelope by radiation. It cannot be transferred between the anode and glass by convection as the tube is evacuated. Some heat is transferred via conduction through the anode stem (this becomes the main process at lower temperatures as heat radiation becomes less significant). From the glass, heat is transferred to the insulating oil and the tube housing by convection.
   b. **False**. It is transferred by radiation and convection.

   c. **True.** Blackening substantially increases the emissivity coefficient.
   d. **True.**
   e. **True.**

19. a. **False.** In a self-rectified tube, electrons travel towards the anode only during the positive half of the waveform. During the negative half of the cycle, the filament has positive potential and does not emit electrons; at high tube currents, the anode may reach temperatures sufficient for thermionic emission and electrons may flow towards the filament, destroying the tube.
   b. **False.** In a half-rectified circuit, the negative half of the voltage waveform is eliminated. As potential across the tube during this period of the cycle is zero, there is no electron flow and no X-ray production.
   c. **False.** In a fully rectified circuit, the negative half of the cycle is 'flipped' into positive. Therefore, in both halves of the cycle, the filament and the target have the correct polarity to produce X-rays. However, the voltage across the tube fluctuates from zero to maximum, and the mean energy of the photons produced is relatively low.
   d. **True.** With three overlapping fully rectified waveforms, the fluctuations in the tube voltage (ripple) are greatly diminished. The voltage across the tube never falls to zero and the efficiency of X-ray production is higher, as is the mean photon energy. High-frequency generators provide yet further improvements with a practically constant potential.
   e. **True.** More filtration is needed to eliminate photons with lower energies produced by the latter.

20. a. **True.**
   b. **False.** Filtration does not affect the maximum energy of the beam spectrum, which is always equal in keV to the tube potential in kV.
   c. **True.** Filtration selectively removes the lower energy photons so it reduces the quantity. It shifts the mean energy of the remaining photons to a higher level, so it increases the beam quality.
   d. **True.**
   e. **False.** The HVL depends on the quality of radiation (energy spectrum), which is not changed by altering mA.

21. a. **True.** They describe the maximal operational settings that are permissible without damage to the anode and tube housing.
   b. **True.** There are rating charts that display curves showing the maximum permissible mA depending on exposure time and peak kV (kVp) for a particular X-ray tube and focal spot size.
   c. **False.** The size of the focal spot has an influence on the tube current that can safely be tolerated.
   d. **True.**
   e. **False.** Ratings for repeated exposures are lower as heat accumulation needs to be taken into account.

22. a. **False.** Depending on examination type, this ratio may vary from 10 (for a PA chest X-ray) to over 5000 (in the case of a lateral lumbar spine radiograph).
    b. **False.** A dose of approximately 3 µGy is required.
    c. **True.**
    d. **False.** With increased kV, the X-ray beam is more penetrating and a lower entrance dose is required to produce the same exit dose. In general, the highest peak kV (kVp) producing acceptable image contrast should be used.
    e. **True.** This is because increasing filtration makes the beam more penetrating.

23. a. **True.** Even though increasing the distance necessitates the increase in mAs, it decreases the skin dose as the beam entering the patient is spread over a larger surface area. It also decreases the dose to deeper tissues to a lesser extent.
    b. **True.** This is due to a reduction of the required exposure factors (less tissue thickness to penetrate) and the amount of scattered radiation.
    c. **True.**
    d. **False.** The exit dose needs to be increased by a factor equal to the Bucky factor of the grid (the ratio of radiation incident on the grid to the transmitted radiation) to obtain the same film exposure.
    e. **False.** Use of an air gap requires a higher tube output and increases the patient dose.

24. a. **True.** There is less scatter in the forward direction and it is less penetrating.
    b. **True.** This reduces the amount of scatter produced.
    c. **True.** This also reduces the amount of scatter produced.
    d. **False.** A grid reduces the amount of scattered radiation reaching the imager, but not the amount of scatter leaving the patient. As it necessitates an increase in tube output, the grid may actually increase the amount of scatter produced (and the patient's dose).
    e. **False.** This is based on the same principle as (d).

25. a. **False.** It does not influence the radiographic contrast.
    b. **True.**
    c. **True.**
    d. **True.**
    e. **True.**

26. a. **True.**
    b. **False.** The line density of a grid (number of lead strips per cm) is usually 30–80 cm^{-1} (typically 40).
    c. **False.** Usually aluminium, carbon fibre or plastic are used as interspace material.
    d. **True.**
    e. **False.** It is typically 8:1. High-ratio grids (12:1–16:1) are used with very large fields and high peak kV (kVp).

27. a. **True.** This means that if the X-ray tube was located at infinity, the incident beam would be parallel to the lead strips and no primary radiation would be lost. With a finite focus-to-film distance, the X-rays towards the periphery of the beam strike the lead strips obliquely and are attenuated (grid cut-off). This is more

pronounced for high grid ratios (therefore parallel grids rarely have ratios higher than 6:1) and short tube-grid distances (therefore parallel grids should not generally be used at distances of less than 150 cm).

b. **True.** In a focused grid, the lead strips are tilted progressively from the centre to the edges, pointing in the direction of a point in space termed the convergent point. If the focal point of the tube is in the convergent point, there is no loss of primary radiation. In practice, there is a degree of latitude with regard to focal point placement – it may be positioned within a range of distances (focusing range) without significant loss of primary radiation. The focusing range is wide for low-ratio grids and narrow for high-ratio grids (the high-ratio grids therefore require more precise positioning).

c. **False.** The resulting ratio is the sum of the individual ratios.

d. **True.** This depends on the grid ratio and factors affecting the amount of scatter produced (e.g. kVp, depth of the patient tissue and field size).

e. **True.** This is because the amount of scatter arising in a small patient is low and the increase in dose caused by the grid would be highly undesirable.

28. a. **True.** It is based on differences in the degree to which different tissues attenuate high- and low-energy photons.

b. **True.** By subtracting images obtained at high and low peak kV (kVp), selective bone and soft tissue images can be obtained.

c. **False.** This is true for dual-exposure systems that obtain two radiographs sequentially at different kVp. There are also single-exposure systems where two image plates divided by a copper filter ('sandwiched detectors') are simultaneously exposed, with the back detector receiving filtered, higher energy photons.

d. **True.**

e. **True.** This is due to a slight (200 ms) time delay between the two exposures.

29. a. **True.**

b. **False.** A slightly higher radiation dose is required.

c. **True.**

d. **True.**

e. **True.** These are the unsubtracted image, the selective soft tissue image and the selective bone image.

30. a. **False.** It is tested using a digital kV meter.

b. **True.**

c. **False.** In the range of 60–120 kV, tube output is proportional to the square of the peak kV (kVp^2). For lower kV (e.g. in mammography), output is proportional to kVp^3.

d. **True.**

e. **False.** It is usually tested every 1–2 months.

Film-screen radiography – Questions

A. K. Yamamoto

1. **Concerning the construction and processing of radiographic film:**
   a. Most films typically have a single layer of emulsion
   b. An emulsion of silver iodide is most commonly used
   c. The grain size of the emulsion is directly related to the speed of the film
   d. Production of the latent image occurs independently of the cation component of the emulsion
   e. Altering the order of the processing of exposed film does not significantly affect the overall image quality

2. **Concerning the properties of radiographic film:**
   a. Optical density is a measure of film blackening based on the degree of transmission of incident light on the film
   b. Using double-sided emulsion has no effect on optical density
   c. The greater the optical density of a film, the lower the intensity of the transmitted light beam
   d. A useful range of optical densities is approximately 0.25–4
   e. Different optical densities in areas within the same film are what produce image contrast when viewing the image

3. **Concerning the properties of radiographic film, with reference to the characteristic curve:**
   a. 'Base plus fog' refers to the optical density of unexposed, undeveloped emulsion
   b. Films with high speed are less sensitive to changes in exposure
   c. Film latitude refers to the range of exposures producing film darkening within the useful optical density range
   d. An increase in film gamma decreases film latitude
   e. Film speed is increased by using double-layered emulsion

4. **Concerning the use of intensifying screens:**
   a. Most radiographic films in clinical practice do not require the use of intensifying screens
   b. Intensifying screens increase the optical density, which may be obtained over a fixed range of exposures
   c. A material that increases the likelihood of Compton scattering should be used for constructing the screen
   d. Intensifying screens are able to convert approximately 50% of X-ray energy into light
   e. Overall image sharpness is not affected by the use of a screen

5. **Concerning the use of grids:**
   a. Grids are always required for adequate production of the radiographic image
   b. Grids increase the mA required to produce an adequately exposed image
   c. A reduction in the grid thickness will increase the amount of scatter that is removed
   d. The grid factor is a measure of how much the grid will affect magnification of the image
   e. Reducing the distance of the patient from the film can help to reduce the effect of scatter

6. **Concerning noise within a radiographic image:**
   a. The level of noise decreases with increased patient dose
   b. The signal-to-noise ratio (SNR) increases with increased patient dose
   c. When imaging tissues with low inherent contrast (such as in mammography), the effect of noise is less significant
   d. When imaging tissues with high inherent contrast, the effect of noise is less significant
   e. The effect of noise can be reduced by using a film with high gamma

7. **Concerning unsharpness within a radiographic image:**
   a. Unsharpness is not affected by the thickness of a film screen
   b. Film-screen unsharpness is generally not important for most X-ray examinations
   c. Crossover contributes more to overall unsharpness than parallax
   d. Geometric unsharpness is decreased by using a smaller focal spot
   e. Geometric unsharpness is increased by decreasing the object-to-film distance

8. **Concerning unsharpness within a radiographic image:**
   a. A shorter exposure time will help reduce movement unsharpness
   b. In the clinical setting, movement unsharpness cannot be significantly reduced
   c. Unsharpness affects the overall spatial resolution of the image
   d. A film with a double layer of emulsion increases unsharpness
   e. Unsharpness is minimized by increased film-screen separation

9. **Factors affecting image quality:**
   a. Increasing the mA will increase the quality of the image
   b. Increasing grain size within the film improves the resolution
   c. Increasing crystal size within a screen decreases the resolution
   d. Increasing crystal size within a screen decreases the dose
   e. Resolution and noise may be altered independently of one another

10. **With regard to factors affecting image quality:**
    a. Increasing the kV decreases the probability of photons interacting within the target
    b. Scattered photons will have less energy at higher peak kV (kVp) values due to greater loss of energy
    c. Increasing kVp means that contrast is improved
    d. The effect on resolution of using a screen with large crystals may be compensated for by using a film with small grains
    e. In practice, it is the film/screen combination that is usually varied rather than the kV

11. **With regard to factors affecting image quality:**
    a. Using a low kV is useful when it is important to keep the radiation dose to a minimum
    b. The latitude describes the dynamic range of the imaging system
    c. Compression may help improve contrast at the expense of increased dose
    d. Unless the mA is increased, the improvement in contrast when using a grid will not be seen
    e. Using a screen with a greater conversion factor while maintaining the mA increases quantum mottle

12. **Concerning factors affecting the entrance surface dose (ESD):**
    a. The orientation of the patient to the film (anterior–posterior (AP) vs lateral) does not alter the ESD
    b. Changes in focus-to-film distance (FFD) do not alter the ESD because changes in mA are required to maintain an adequate film dose
    c. Increasing the kV reduces the ESD, assuming mA is constant
    d. Filtration reduces the patient dose by decreasing the likelihood of the Compton effect
    e. Unintentional absorption of X-rays after they have already passed through the tissue will not affect the ESD, assuming mA is constant

13. **Concerning quality assurance in film-screen radiography:**
    a. It requires a check of every exposure to ensure that it is adequate
    b. Quality assurance is not covered in legislation, although good practice demands that it be enforced
    c. Regulations are in place that dictate what test should be performed
    d. Quality assurance tests generally have cut-off levels at which equipment should not be used
    e. Sensitometry may be used to test the performance of a film-screen system

14. **Concerning quality assurance in film-screen radiography:**
    a. It is insufficient to test only the film speed and contrast index
    b. A gradual change in the speed of the film is more likely to be related to problems during the processing of film than to problems with the film batch
    c. Screens should be changed routinely at yearly intervals
    d. The tube potential may be tested by assessing the kV of the X-ray beam
    e. X-ray output should increase with increasing kV

15. **Concerning quality assurance in film-screen radiography:**
    a. The testing of filtration within the system is not routinely performed
    b. Total filtration should be equivalent to at least 1.5 mm of aluminium
    c. Assessment of optical density is the main measure of correct automatic exposure control (AEC) functioning
    d. Focal spot size may be estimated using the pinhole method
    e. A lower-than-expected output dose measurement is unrelated to exposure time

16. **Concerning intensifying screens:**
    a. They typically measure 1 cm in thickness
    b. They are usually made of calcium tungstate phosphor

43

c. They convert the pattern of X-ray intensities into one of light, which is detected by the film
d. Films and screens should be matched
e. A phosphor with a K-edge value similar to the mean photon energy should be selected

17. Concerning developing conditions:
   a. Decreasing the temperature of the developer increases the film speed
   b. Increasing the temperature of the developer increases the fog level
   c. Increasing the development time reduces the fog level
   d. Decreasing the developer concentration reduces the fog level
   e. Increasing the developer concentration or developing time will increase the film speed

18. Concerning linear tomography:
   a. It is able to clearly demonstrate structures at various depths within the patient in the same image
   b. It is able to reduce the effect of superimposition of structures within the image
   c. It relies on the simultaneous movement of the X-ray tube and patient
   d. Increasing the tomographic angle increases the thickness of the cut
   e. Section thickness decreases as the distance from the pivot to the film increases

19. Concerning linear tomography:
   a. The thickness of the plane in focus may be in the order of several mm
   b. The level of the imaged plane within the patient is altered by raising or lowering the pivot position
   c. Blurring increases with decreasing distance from the focal plane
   d. The tomographic angle is usually in the order of 40°
   e. Contrast is improved by imaging thin slices

20. Concerning resolution within the image:
   a. Spatial resolution is the ability to distinguish adjacent objects as being separate
   b. Spatial resolution may be measured in line pairs mm^{-1}
   c. The spatial resolution of X-ray films is less than that of an image intensifier
   d. The spatial resolution of X-ray films is greater than that of computed tomography
   e. Spatial resolution may be determined by the properties of the radiographic film

21. Duplitized (two layers of emulsion) radiographic films:
   a. Reduce the radiation dose to produce an adequate image
   b. Increase the fog level
   c. May take longer to process
   d. Have increased scatter compared with a film with a single layer of emulsion
   e. Are less expensive to manufacture than film with a single layer of emulsion

22. Concerning silver halide emulsion:
   a. It is the halide that donates electrons when irradiated
   b. It provides silver atoms for conversion to silver ions

c. It is unaffected by fixing agents during processing
d. It is insensitive to visible light
e. It consists of silver combined with one of the halogen elements

23. An air gap:
    a. Describes the distance between the patient and the X-ray focus
    b. Reduces contrast
    c. Reduces the dose
    d. Will cause magnification of the final image
    e. Is an alternative to using a grid

24. Scatter may be reduced by:
    a. Tissue compression
    b. Increasing the kV
    c. Increasing the distance between the patient and the film
    d. Placing a grid between the X-ray focus and the patient
    e. Using collimation

25. Concerning grids:
    a. They may be focused or unfocused
    b. They may produce artefacts on the final image
    c. Stationary grids are commonly employed
    d. The higher the grid factor, the greater the exposure required to produce a film of the same radiographic density
    e. The effect of grids on scatter depends mainly on the grid ratio

26. Concerning screens:
    a. The intensification factor (IF) describes the reduction in exposure when using a screen
    b. Using smaller crystals increases the screen speed
    c. The IF is not directly related to the kV
    d. Screen speed is related to the conversion efficiency of the phosphor
    e. Screen speed is decreased with the rare earth metals

27. The following improve contrast:
    a. Collimation
    b. A higher kV
    c. Reduced beam filtration (for a given kV)
    d. Films with higher gamma
    e. The use of contrast media

28. Concerning entrance surface doses (ESDs) in adults (national diagnostic reference levels, 2007)
    a. Chest posterior–anterior (PA) radiograph = 0.2 mGy
    b. Abdominal radiograph = 2 mGy
    c. A lumbar spine anterior–posterior (AP) radiograph is greater than a pelvis AP radiograph

    d. Imaging the vertebral column typically requires a greater dose for the AP view compared with the lateral (LAT) view

    e. A LAT view of the skull is greater than a PA view

29. Factors that reduce the dose to the patient include:

    a. Increased filtration

    b. Reduced collimation

    c. Using a grid with paediatric patients

    d. Using an intensifying screen

    e. Increasing the X-ray focus-to-patient distance

30. Increasing the tube potential:

    a. Improves film contrast

    b. Increases the dose to the patient

    c. Reduces the exposure time

    d. Increases geometric unsharpness

    e. Has no effect on motion unsharpness

Film-screen radiography – Answers

1. a. **False.** Most films usually have a double layer of emulsion attached to a polyester film base. This allows increased speed as two intensifying screens can be used. Mammography films usually are single-layered.
   b. **False.** Silver bromide is most commonly used.
   c. **True.** The larger the grain size, the faster the film. Larger grains provide a larger target for the light photons and so fewer photons are required to produce the image.
   d. **False.** Both the anion (bromide) and cation (silver) are required to produce the latent image: the bromide is the electron donor and the silver ion becomes deposited and later converted to the black silver atom to produce the image.
   e. **False.** Post-processing is vital in converting the latent image to a visible image. This requires the conversion of silver ions to visible silver atoms (electron gain) from electron donors (e.g. phenidone and hydroquinone), a process known as film development. Unexposed grains also need to be removed from the film (to render the film stable in light) and the process of development halted to prevent fogging, a process known as fixing.

2. a. **True.** Optical density $= \log_{10} Io/In$, where Io is the intensity of incident light and In is the intensity of transmitted light.
   b. **False.** The optical densities for each layer are cumulative so that, for the same level of exposure, the densities are increased compared with using a single layer.
   c. **True.** Referring back to the equation in (a), if the optical density $= 1$, then only 10% of light is transmitted, as $\log_{10} 10 = 1$. Likewise, if optical density $= 2$, then only 1% of light is transmitted ($\log_{10} 100 = 2$).
   d. **False.** Optical densities of around 2 may be seen with normal illumination; however, an optical density of 3 appears very dark and requires the use of a focal bright light to see through it. An optical density of 4 means that only 1/10,000 of the incident light has been transmitted, so the film will appear black.
   e. **True.** Contrast may be measured as the difference in optical densities: $OD_1 - OD_2$. This difference will be produced by the nature of the tissue being imaged.

3. a. **False.** This refers to the inherent optical density of the film material plus unexposed developed emulsion. This should be less than 0.2. However, film that has been stored for too long a period or at too high a temperature may have higher values, in which case it should not be used.
   b. **False.** Film speed is a measure of film sensitivity when exposed, i.e. a high-speed film requires less exposure to produce a certain optical density than a film of low speed.

c. **True.** Films with narrow latitude require a smaller range of exposures to achieve darkening over the useful optical density range, i.e. they provide good contrast between tissues. Wide-latitude films are the reverse, requiring a greater range of exposures to achieve this range.

d. **True.** Film gamma refers to the slope of the linear part of the characteristic curve and is the ratio of the differences between optical density and film exposure at two given points on the slope. If gamma increases, then film latitude decreases and contrast increases. These are inherent properties of any given film.

e. **True.** The optical densities for each layer are cumulative so that, for a given exposure, the total optical densities will be greater than using a single layer. This assumes that the total thickness of emulsion is doubled.

4. a. **False.** This is only true for dental films. Most films do require intensifying screens for image acquisition, and this acts to reduce the radiation dose required by 30–300-fold.

b. **True.** They increase not only the gradient of the characteristic curve (film gamma), but also the speed of the film.

c. **False.** Ideally a material that increases the likelihood of photoelectric absorption (which is related to the cube of the atomic number (Z^3)) should be used. Materials such as tungsten or rare earth metals are selected (lanthanum, $Z = 57$, and gadolinium, $Z = 64$).

d. **False.** The actual value is much lower, in the region of 10–15% for the earth metals and less than 5% for calcium tungstate.

e. **False.** Overall image sharpness is particularly affected when thicker screens are used, as the light rays produced within the screen are able to travel over a further distance and in different directions before reaching the film. This also means that the light may be absorbed before reaching the film. This effect can be minimized by using two thinner screens with double-sided film.

5. a. **False.** Grids are useful as they help to reduce the effect of scatter and improve the quality of the image and so are generally used. However, in some settings, a grid is not used when the effect of scatter is reduced (e.g. when there is less tissue for the photons to travel through, such as during paediatric imaging).

b. **True.** As some photons are blocked from reaching the radiographic film, a greater dose will be required to produce the same optical density of the film than if a grid was not used.

c. **False.** This change will decrease the amount of scatter that is removed. Increasing the distance between each of the lead grid strips will also have the same effect. The ratio of the thickness, h, and the horizontal distance between the strips, d, form the grid ratio = h/d. Hence, grids with higher grid ratios are more effective at removing scatter.

d. **False.** A grid will have no effect on magnification. The grid factor indicates the increase in exposure (and hence dose) that is required when a grid is used compared with not using a grid.

e. **False.** Increasing the object-to-film distance can help to reduce scatter. This is known as an air gap and helps reduce scatter by the principle of the inverse square law. It can act as an alternative to using a grid.

6. a. **False**. Noise will increase as a proportion of the number of photons (n) that are detected in the image (as noise $= \sqrt{n}$).
   b. **True**. Although the amount of noise will increase with increasing patient dose, the actual SNR increases and so improves image quality.
   c. **False**. Noise is more significant. Differentiating between the nature of soft-tissue structures is more important when there is less inherent contrast within the tissues being imaged. Therefore, noise will prevent this differentiation.
   d. **True**.
   e. **False**. The higher film gamma produces more radiographic contrast within the film for the same exposure, but also has the same effect on the noise, which is displayed in the image.

7. a. **False**. X-rays produce light photons within the screen, which can then spread out in all directions and so decrease the unsharpness. This effect will be increased if a thicker screen is used, as there is a greater distance over which the light photon can travel.
   b. **False**. This depends on what is being imaged. It becomes less important when imaging thicker sections of the body or regions where fine detail is less important, e.g. radiograph of the pelvis. When imaging extremities with a requirement for fine detail, a thinner screen is used (although this will require an increased dose for the same optical density).
   c. **True**. The use of double-sided screens with double film has the added advantages of overcoming the use of a single thicker screen and the cumulative effect of optical densities, but introduces the problem of crossover where the light from one screen produces an image in the opposite emulsion and vice versa. Parallax may contribute to unsharpness if the image is viewed obliquely (which is often not the case).
   d. **True**. A small focal spot decreases the size of the penumbra at the edge of the image.
   e. **False**. Decreasing the object-to-film distance reduces the size of the penumbra. Increasing the distance between the focal spot and the object also decreases geometric unsharpness. These three variables are connected by the equation:

$$\text{Geometric unsharpness} = \frac{(\text{focal spot size}) \times (\text{object} - \text{film distance})}{(\text{focal spot} - \text{film distance}) - (\text{object} - \text{film distance})}$$

8. a. **True**. However, this will be at the expense of requiring a higher mA.
   b. **False**. This may be achieved in two ways. Firstly, by immobilization of the target, as is performed with mammography where definition of structures is of increased importance. Secondly, by performing radiographs during breath holding, which minimizes the effects of respiration.
   c. **True**. The three main sources of unsharpness (screen, geometric and movement) all affect the resolution of the image (resolution is the overall ability within the imaging system to detect two objects separately from one another).
   d. **False**. This assumes that the overall thickness of the emulsion has not increased but is split equally between the two layers.
   e. **False**. Close opposition of the film and screen is a requirement to minimize unsharpness.

9. a. **True.** Increasing the mA increases the signal-to-noise ratio (SNR) at the expense of increasing the patient dose.
   b. **False.** Larger grains mean less are present within a certain volume so it therefore becomes more difficult to distinguish changes in optical density over a certain area.
   c. **True.** Larger crystals will emit more photons, which have the potential to travel in multiple directions before reaching the film. This will increase the unsharpness within the image.
   d. **True.** Larger crystals will emit more light photons than a screen of the same thickness with smaller crystals (this holds true if the fluorescent material of the two screens is the same and has the same conversion factor).
   e. **True.** Decreasing crystal size within the screen will improve the resolution but decrease the SNR within the image. However, this may be overcome by increasing the dose.

10. a. **True.** The probability of the photoelectric effect decreases with the cube of the photon energy. Compton scatter does not change significantly with increasing photon energy.
    b. **False.** Overall, they will still have more energy.
    c. **False.** Using a greater kVp means the scattered photons have more energy and are more likely to reach the film, which will reduce the contrast. In addition, if the intended absorption by the tissues being imaged is reduced due to reduced photoelectric effect, this will also reduce the contrast within the image.
    d. **False.** Resolution is affected most by the part of the imaging system that demonstrates limited resolution.
    e. **False.** kV is one of the three main variables that is changed to influence image quality (mA and exposure time being the other two).

11. a. **False.** Although the dose should always be kept to a minimum level, sufficient to make the test adequate, a low kV is used when it is important to achieve sufficient contrast, e.g. for mammography (note that this then requires a higher entrance surface dose than if a higher kV was used).
    b. **True.**
    c. **False.** Compression will improve the contrast by reducing scatter, but also reduces the dose as the tissues are less thick, increasing radiation transmission.
    d. **True.** Although a grid will remove scattered radiation and so improve contrast, it will also remove unscattered radiation. This will lead to a reduction in optical density and, unless this is compensated for by increasing the mA, this benefit will not be seen.
    e. **False.** The overall number of photons is increased due to the greater conversion factor of the screen. Therefore, the signal-to-noise ratio is increased.

12. a. **False.** The ESD will need to increase to ensure adequate transmission of the X-ray photons as the thickness of the tissue being imaged increases to produce a satisfactory image. Other factors that may also influence this will depend on the nature of the tissue being imaged, e.g. an AP lumbar spine image requires a greater dose than an AP thoracic spine image.

b. **False.** Although the mA must be increased as the FFD is increased, there is an overall reduction in the ESD due to the relationship of X-ray intensity to distance being an inverse square law.

c. **False.** Increasing the photon energy means that the beam is more penetrating and more photons will reach the image receptor. Therefore, the ESD may be reduced but only if mA is reduced concurrently.

d. **False.** It reduces the patient dose by removing those low-energy photons that would not have contributed to the image (and would just be absorbed by the tissue). This is due to a reduction of the photoelectric effect rather than the Compton effect, which is constant at all photon energies.

e. **True.** However, the image quality will be affected as a consequence.

13. a. **False.** Quality assurance is a system that tries to ensure, by having a system of checks in place, that an adequate image is obtained. However, this does not require every exposure to be assessed.

b. **False.** It constitutes part of the Ionising Radiation Regulations (IRR) 1999.

c. **False.** The regulations state that quality assurance should be performed, rather than what the actual test should be.

d. **True.**

e. **True.** This measures optical densities at various repeatable exposure settings. If the densities produced are outside a certain range, this indicates that image quality may be compromised.

14. a. **True.** The base plus fog level and maximum density (D_{max}) also need to be tested. These may be affected by long-term storage of the film at incorrect temperatures.

b. **True.**

c. **False.** There is no set time as to when they need to be changed. When the sensitivity of a screen has reduced by 20%, then generally it should be changed. This may be tested by producing test films at set kV and mAs values and comparing the optical density produced.

d. **True.** Although the tube potential is not usually measured directly, an electronic meter may be used to demonstrate the kV and its variation with the exposure time using an oscilloscope.

e. **True.**

15. a. **False.** The amount of filtration is most important when the diagnostic information depends on fine contrast being demonstrated between the tissues being imaged (e.g. in mammography). This contrast may be lost if there is beam hardening if filtration is too great.

b. **False.** It should be equivalent to 2.5 mm of aluminium.

c. **True.** The AEC functions by terminating the exposure once a film has a received dose sufficient to produce an adequate film. Therefore, the optical density of test films can be monitored as the level at which the AEC is set and then varied while monitoring the dose. Test subject thickness (usually Perspex) may also be altered at the same time.

   d. **True.** This technique produces a magnified image of the focal spot. The focal spot size can then be calculated by determining the magnification by knowing the focus-to-film and pinhole-to-film distances.

   e. **False.** Along with changing the tube potential and tube current, a shorter exposure time may also reduce the output.

16. a. **False.** The thickness is much less, usually 1–2 mm.
   b. **False.** They are usually made of the rare earth metals such as gadolinium oxysulphide or lanthanum oxybromide.
   c. **True.** To produce an image on film without a screen would require high levels of radiation due to its relative insensitivity. Screens are used to reduce the dose required to produce an adequate image.
   d. **True.** The colour of the emitted light will vary depending on the phosphor used within the screen. The film should therefore be sensitive to the emitted light to ensure that the image is obtained. For example, gadolinium oxysulphide emits green light, whereas lanthanum oxybromide emits blue light.
   e. **True.** This ensures that there is increased attenuation of the radiation spectrum, whose intensity may then be converted into one of light and thus represented as an image on the radiographic film.

17. a. **False.** It decreases film speed.
   b. **True.**
   c. **False.** It increases the fog level by developing unexposed grains.
   d. **True.**
   e. **True.**

18. a. **False.** It is only able to demonstrate structures within a selected slice at any one time.
   b. **True.** The structures located above and below the selected slice are deliberately blurred out. The structures within the selected slice are sharply imaged. This is in contrast to conventional film-screen radiography where all structures within the direction of the X-ray beam appear superimposed on another (e.g. a chest radiograph with ribs, soft tissue and lung all appearing in the same image).
   c. **False.** The patient remains fixed in position. It is the cassette tray and X-ray tube that move in opposite directions to one another.
   d. **False.** Decreasing the angle increases the thickness of the cut. When the tomographic angle is zero, the image would be the same as an anterior–posterior radiograph.
   e. **True.**

19. a. **True.**
   b. **True.**
   c. **False.** It is those structures closest to the focal plane that are most sharply imaged.
   d. **True.**
   e. **False.** Contrast is reduced.

20. a. **True.**
   b. **True.**

  c. **False.** It is much greater (e.g. 2–4 line pairs mm^{-1} for fluoroscopy compared with more than 10 line pairs mm^{-1} with X-ray films).

  d. **True.**

  e. **True.**

21. a. **True.** This assumes that the overall thickness of the emulsion is doubled.

  b. **False.**

  c. **True.** It may take longer for the processing substances to penetrate all the emulsion, if the overall total emulsion thickness has increased.

  d. **False.** It has no effect.

  e. **False.**

22. a. **True.**

  b. **False.** The reverse is true: the silver ions are converted to atoms, which provide the blackness within the final image.

  c. **False.**

  d. **False.**

  e. **True.**

23. a. **False.** It is the distance between the patient and the film.

  b. **False.** It improves contrast by reducing the amount of scattered radiation that is able to reach the film.

  c. **False.** As less of the primary radiation reaches the film (as a result of the inverse square law), this requires an increase in the kV/mA to compensate.

  d. **True.**

  e. **True.**

24. a. **True.** There is less tissue that can act to scatter the radiation.

  b. **False.** Increasing the kV means that any scattered radiation is more penetrating and may reach the film.

  c. **True.** This is known as an air gap.

  d. **False.** Although grids are used to reduce scatter, they are placed between the patient and the film.

  e. **True.** This reduces the amount of tissue being irradiated and so reduces scatter.

25. a. **True.** This describes the orientation of the lead strips in relation to the path of the X-ray beam. As X-rays are divergent from their source, focused grids have their strips tilted to allow more of the primary radiation to pass through the grid.

  b. **True.** Shadows from the lead strips may be superimposed on the final image.

  c. **False.** As described above, shadows may be projected onto the final image. This effect may be reduced by using moving grids, which oscillate during the exposure. These are more commonly used than stationary grids.

  d. **True.** This is a ratio of the exposures required with and without a grid.

  e. **True.** The grid ratio describes the effect of the grid in reducing scatter. The higher the grid ratio, the more scatter will be removed.

26. a. **True**. It is a ratio of the exposure without a screen compared with the exposure with a screen.
    b. **False**. It decreases the screen speed.
    c. **True**. It is a property of the screen.
    d. **True**. A better conversion efficiency will increase the speed.
    e. **False**. It is increased, as they have K-edges, which are in the spectrum of the mean photon energy, thus increasing the photoelectric effect.

27. a. **True**. Collimation improves contrast by reducing scatter.
    b. **False**. Higher kV means there is more scatter and less difference in absorption between tissues.
    c. **True**. This is due to a reduction of the overall mean energy of the X-ray beam.
    d. **True**.
    e. **True**.

28. a. **True**.
    b. **False**. It is 6 mGy.
    c. **True**. (6 mGy versus 4 mGy).
    d. **False**. The reverse is true and is related to the amount of tissue that the X-ray beam needs to pass through.
    e. **False**. The skull has a greater sagittal length than coronal length.

Guidance on the establishment and use of diagnostic reference levels (DRLs) (Department of Health, April 2007): national DRLs for individual radiographs on adult patients. AP, anterior-posterior; PA, posterior-anterior; LAT, lateral.

Radiograph	ESD per radiograph (mGy)	Dose–area product (DAP) per radiograph (Gy cm^2)
Skull AP or PA	3	–
Skull LAT	1.5	–
Chest PA	0.2	0.12
Chest LAT	1.0	–
Thoracic spine AP	3.5	–
Thoracic spine LAT	10	–
Lumbar spine AP	6	1.6
Lumbar spine LAT	14	3
Abdomen AP	6	3
Pelvis AP	4	3

29. a. **True.**
  b. **False.** Better collimation prevents unnecessary exposure to tissues and also acts to reduce scatter.
  c. **False.** As younger patients are smaller, a lower kV may be used and so scatter will be less and grids can be avoided. Because grids reduce the intensity of the main radiation beam, a grid will result in an increased dose to the patient by increasing the required mA.
  d. **True.**
  e. **True.** However, this can lead to a reduction in magnification.

30. a. **False.** It decreases film contrast by reducing the probability of photoelectric absorption in tissues and increasing the scattered radiation contributing to the final image.
  b. **False.** The beam is more penetrating; therefore, less radiation is required to produce an adequate image.
  c. **True.**
  d. **False.** It has no effect.
  e. **False.** Using a higher kV reduces the required exposure time so it can indirectly reduce motion unsharpness.

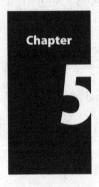

Chapter

5

Digital radiography – Questions

A. K. Yamamoto

1. Concerning a digital radiography system:
   a. An early step in image acquisition is conversion of data from an analogue to digital format
   b. The size of the image detector is not important, as the final image may be manipulated electronically
   c. Detector sensitivity must be high
   d. Pixel size influences image resolution
   e. Noise is less significant than with film-screen radiography

2. The requirements of a digital radiography system are:
   a. Good X-ray sensitivity
   b. A small field size
   c. A digital-to-analogue converter (DAC)
   d. A narrow dynamic range
   e. A locally based archive

3. Concerning the digital radiographic image:
   a. It is represented numerically in digital form
   b. The image is divided into a matrix consisting of multiple pixels
   c. The greater the sampling frequency, the greater the spatial resolution
   d. Decreasing the detector sampling frequency may reduce detector sensitivity
   e. The image may be read out directly from the detector electronically

4. Concerning the digital radiographic image:
   a. Signal digitization expresses the image as continuous grey-scale values
   b. The function of the analogue-to-digital converter (ADC) is to digitize the input while maintaining resolution of the information
   c. A binary system is used for signal digitization
   d. Eight bits is typically sufficient for most images
   e. Data compression for storage may lead to loss of data

5. The number of bytes of a digital image is dependent upon:
   a. The number of pixels within the image
   b. Pixel size, assuming matrix size is constant
   c. The magnification of the image
   d. The bit size per pixel
   e. The sampling frequency, assuming receptor size is constant

6. Concerning image acquisition in computed radiography:
   a. It depends on fluorescence within the X-ray screen
   b. An image plate is used
   c. The equipment chosen will depend on the degree of resolution required
   d. The latent image is stored by electrons located within the valence bands of the phosphor
   e. It requires electrons to return to their resting state for the image to be obtained

7. Concerning the computed radiography image plate:
   a. A laser input is required to erase residual signal from the image plate
   b. It reduces the generation of scatter
   c. It may be used for tomography
   d. Unprocessed image plates will retain the latent image
   e. It has a narrow dynamic range

8. Concerning signal processing with computed radiography:
   a. The signal-to-dose relationship differs from that of film-screen radiography
   b. Contrast within the final computed radiography image may be greater than is achievable with film-screen radiography
   c. It demonstrates better spatial resolution than film-screen radiography
   d. Increasing pixel size improves resolution
   e. Image plate processing does not affect resolution

9. Concerning the modulation transfer function (MTF):
   a. The MTF relates to the ability of the digital imaging system to demonstrate spatial resolution within the final image
   b. The lower the MTF, the greater the spatial resolution demonstrated
   c. The MTF of a detail film-screen system is greater at higher spatial frequencies than for a computed radiography system
   d. The typical limiting spatial resolution of a computed radiography system is 5 line pairs mm^{-1}
   e. High-resolution computed radiography systems may achieve an MTF of 1.5

10. Concerning artefacts in computed radiography:
    a. A ghost image refers to inadequate exposure of the image plate
    b. Artefacts from stationary grids do not occur
    c. Artefacts may be related to incorrect imaging processing techniques
    d. Laser-stimulated emission may be contributory
    e. Repeat exposures are not required for artefact correction

11. Concerning noise in computed radiography:
    a. It has a similar effect on image quality as in film-screen radiography
    b. It is unrelated to the type of image plate used
    c. It is unrelated to the patient dose
    d. Edge enhancement increases noise
    e. It may be reduced by low-pass spatial filtering

12. Concerning computed radiography image acquisition:
    a. The detective quantum efficiency (DQE) is a measure of how efficiently the detector records information within the X-ray beam
    b. The DQE for some computed radiography systems approaches 1
    c. The greater the resolution of the image plate, the greater the DQE
    d. The DQE is increased with dual-read image plates
    e. Improved DQE can lead to a reduction in patient dose

13. Concerning the exposure index in computed radiography:
    a. The exposure index is a measure of the dose incident on the image plate
    b. The exposure index varies among different manufacturers
    c. Doubling the dose doubles the resulting exposure index
    d. Knowledge of typical exposure indices can help identify overexposures
    e. The exposure index depends solely on the dose given

14. Concerning flat-panel digital radiography:
    a. It is still dependent on separate exposure and readout stages
    b. It requires the use of a silicon-based transistor
    c. Indirect conversion digital receptors are dependent on a scintillator for image acquisition
    d. The X-ray absorption efficiency of indirect digital receptors is less than with computed radiography
    e. An indirect conversion digital receptor is dependent on the conversion of light into electrical charge

15. Concerning indirect conversion digital radiography:
    a. It typically uses a fixed-size detector
    b. It has a digital quantum efficiency (DQE) greater than that with computed radiography image plates
    c. It typically has a radiographic speed of less than 400
    d. It differs from direct conversion detectors due to the use of an X-ray scintillator
    e. It has a resolution of approximately 3–4 line pairs mm^{-1}

16. Concerning the construction of direct conversion detectors:
    a. The photoconductor produces electrical charge when irradiated
    b. It is still dependent on a silicon-based transistor
    c. A potential difference is applied across the photoconductor to increase the charge formed per X-ray photon
    d. The signal for image formation is carried by the negative charge (electrons)
    e. It is designed to be compatible with more than one radiographic machine

17. Which of the following are true regarding the differences between indirect and direct conversion detectors?
    a. The detective quantum efficiency (DQE) of direct conversion detectors is greater than that of indirect conversion detectors
    b. The difference in DQE is due to the difference in the K-edges of caesium iodide and selenium

   c. Lower patient doses are possible with direct than with indirect conversion detectors

   d. For the same patient dose, a greater signal-to-noise ratio is possible with indirect than with direct detectors

   e. Spatial resolution is greater with direct than indirect conversion detectors

18. Which of the following are true regarding the differences between computed and digital radiography?
   a. The detective quantum efficiency (DQE) is greater with digital radiography than with computed radiography
   b. The patient dose may be less with digital radiography than with computed radiography
   c. Spatial resolution is greater with digital radiography than with computed radiography
   d. Initial costs are greater with computed radiography
   e. Both demonstrate a wide dynamic range

19. Regarding the post-processing of digital radiography images:
   a. Irregular shading across the image field is an irreversible artefact
   b. Defective pixels within the matrix may not alter the final image quality
   c. The wide dynamic range of unprocessed data can result in loss of image quality
   d. Auto-ranging is operator dependent
   e. Auto-ranging improves spatial resolution

20. Concerning digital enhancement:
   a. Digital enhancement may be operator-dependent
   b. Grey-scale modification can be used to improve spatial resolution
   c. Grey-scale modification uses a look-up table (LUT) technique
   d. Unsharp masking can help distinguish fine detail within the image
   e. Unsharp masking may increase noise

21. Concerning the display of digital images:
   a. The cathode ray tube is dependent on a scanning photon beam
   b. Over time, cathode ray tubes reliably maintain image quality
   c. Liquid crystal displays (LCDs) exploit variations in light polarization within the crystal for image visualization
   d. Once the image is digitized, it is not possible to view it as a hard copy
   e. Image reproduction is less reliable with flat-panel monitors than with cathode ray tubes

22. Regarding the image associated with digital radiography:
   a. A good-quality image may amount to over 10 Mb of data
   b. Images of a smaller matrix size will tolerate greater compression than images with a larger matrix size
   c. An image detector based on a charge-coupled device (CCD) photosensor is an alternative to the thin-film transistor
   d. Digital radiography uses smaller matrix sizes than are used in computed tomography
   e. The image may be saved as a JPEG

23. Concerning picture archiving and communications systems (PACS):
    a. PACS eliminate the need for film storage
    b. Their correct use is guided by the Data Protection Act (1998)
    c. Primary diagnostic clinical interpretation generally should not be performed from any workstation
    d. Images cannot be accessed simultaneously from different locations
    e. Data compression can help reduce the storage requirements associated with PACS

24. Concerning picture archiving and communications systems (PACS):
    a. Typically, only one archive is used for image storage
    b. The PACS workflow manager is responsible for the retrieval of images from the archive
    c. For effective functioning, PACS requires connection with the hospital information systems (HIS)
    d. PACS is dependent on the HL7 standard for information transfer from the hospital information system
    e. The cost savings compared with hard-copy storage are definite

25. Concerning the Digital Imaging and Communications in Medicine (DICOM) service:
    a. It functions to keep the image file along with the corresponding patient identifying data as separate
    b. It allows medical imaging devices from different manufacturers to be used with a single PACS
    c. The 'modality worklist' service may increase the risk of data input errors
    d. The 'modality push/pull' service allows image storage and retrieval to and from PACS
    e. The 'modality performed procedure step' service provides information about the status of an examination

26. Concerning quality assurance in digital radiography:
    a. Post-imaging processing removes the requirement for quality assurance
    b. There are no guidelines for the recommended specification of the display device required for diagnostic reporting
    c. Image display devices should undergo resolution and grey-scale contrast ratio monitoring every 3 months
    d. Suboptimal images may be restricted on PACS from general clinical viewing until they have been quality assured
    e. The consistent presentation of images is implemented using the grey-scale standard display function (GSDF)

27. When comparing film-screen and digital image receptors, film-screen radiography:
    a. Has a narrower latitude
    b. Has a higher spatial resolution
    c. Separates acquisition and display into separate steps
    d. Has a greater detective quantum efficiency (DQE)
    e. Generally requires a greater radiation dose for the same exposure

28. Concerning digital and computed radiography imaging systems:
    a. They have a similar dynamic range
    b. They are both unaffected by random noise
    c. With an analogue-to-digital converter (ADC), insufficient bits do not affect signal coding
    d. Digital and computed radiography imaging systems benefit from a reduction in image acquisition time compared with film-screen radiography
    e. Computer-aided detection (CAD) may be employed with digital images

29. Regarding spatial resolution in computed and digital imaging systems:
    a. It is affected in indirect digital systems by the spread of light photons within the scintillator
    b. It is unaffected in digital radiography by the size of the detector elements within the thin-film transistor
    c. In computed radiography, spatial resolution is unrelated to the thickness of the phosphor
    d. For both computed and digital radiography, pixel size affects spatial resolution
    e. The modulation transfer function (MTF) is an objective measure of spatial resolution

30. Concerning digital radiography:
    a. It does not require the use of an anti-scatter grid
    b. Fixed system noise may be reduced by post-processing
    c. Detector artefacts may occur as a result of variations in image receptor sensitivity
    d. Automatic exposure control is not used with digital radiography
    e. It requires specific post-processing parameters for paediatric patients

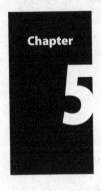

Digital radiography – Answers

1. a. **True.** The image from the detector is converted by the analogue-to-digital converter (ADC) into a digital format before being transferred to the computer system.
   b. **False.** Unlike film-screen radiography where the size of the film can be changed depending on the examination, the detector in digital radiography must be large enough to cover the range of examinations that will be performed on the same system.
   c. **True.** This is to ensure that minimal doses are required.
   d. **True.**
   e. **False.** Noise occurs in all imaging systems and contributes to the final image quality.

2. a. **True.**
   b. **False.** A large field size is required.
   c. **False.** As the image display is usually in a digital format (such as a liquid crystal display (LCD)), conversion back to an analogue signal is not required.
   d. **False.** A wide dynamic range is required to cover the range of exposures that will be necessary when performing a range of different examinations.
   e. **True.**

3. a. **True.**
   b. **True.** A pixel has an assigned value, which represents the signal intensity within the corresponding part of the image. The matrix size refers to the total number of pixels.
   c. **True.**
   d. **False.** Increasing the detector sampling frequency will reduce sensitivity. This is due to a decrease in the relative proportion of the pixel that is sensitive to image detection (known as the 'fill factor').
   e. **True.** In solid-state designs of detector, the micro-circuitry may be integrated with the X-ray absorption layer.

4. a. **False.** They are expressed as discrete grey-scale values. It is the analogue input that is continuous.
   b. **True.**
   c. **True.**
   d. **False.** Eight bits may be sufficient for images with high noise (e.g. radionuclide imaging), but for imaging requiring greater resolution, 12 bits or more are required.
   e. **True.** Greater compression can lead to loss of data (using 'irreversible algorithms').

5. a. **True.**
   b. **False.**
   c. **False.**
   d. **True.**
   e. **True.** Data content increases due to an increase in matrix size.

6. a. **False.** It depends on photo-stimulated phosphorescence. Fluorescence describes the emission of light immediately after the phosphor is exposed to X-rays, while phosphorescence describes delayed emission, which is the property exploited in computed radiography.
   b. **True.** This is the name for the screen comprising barium fluorohalide crystals (halogen elements of bromine, iodine and chlorine) with europium ions, which are usually embedded in a light-reflective layer.
   c. **True.** High-resolution image plates are designed with a thinner layer of phosphor crystals without a light-reflective layer. The compromise with these plates is that they will require a higher dose to obtain an adequate image.
   d. **False.** Electrons located in 'electron traps' within the phosphor store the latent image. These represent energy levels, which differ from those in which the electrons usually exist (the valence bands) prior to irradiation.
   e. **True.**

7. a. **False.** The laser provides energy in the form of red light to allow electrons to return to the conduction band within the phosphor resulting in the emission of energy (in the form of blue light). It is this light that is then detected and converted into a signal.
   b. **False.** The method in which the image is acquired does not affect the generation of scatter.
   c. **True.**
   d. **True.** However, the image will decay over time if unprocessed, as the excited electrons return to their resting state.
   e. **False.** The plates are able to record a much greater range of photon intensity than is possible with film-screen radiography.

8. a. **True.** The relationship differs from the characteristic curve of conventional radiography. Essentially, the response demonstrates wide latitude.
   b. **True.** Even though the computed radiography response demonstrates wide latitude, post-processing of the data may allow better contrast to be seen within the image. This may include rejection of signals outside the useful range and edge enhancement.
   c. **False.**
   d. **False.** The opposite is true.
   e. **False.** The laser light, which is used for processing of the latent image, may be spread out over the phosphor, increasing the area over which light is emitted. This effect is increased with increasing size of the phosphor crystals. The diameter of the laser beam also affects resolution.

9. a. **True.**
   b. **False.** The greater the MTF, the greater the spatial resolution demonstrated. The MTF is a ratio of the output and input modulation of the signal, and generally

decreases as the frequency of the signal increases, i.e. as the MTF approaches zero, then this will be the maximum spatial frequency of that particular system (limiting spatial resolution).

c. **True.**

d. **True.**

e. **False.** As the MTF is a ratio of output:input, its maximum value can never be greater than 1.

10. a. **False.** This is when the image plate has been incompletely erased since the previous exposure.

b. **False.** Grids may be used in computed radiography as in film-screen radiography with the same effect on resultant image quality.

c. **True.** For example, applying incorrect parameters involved in analysis of the intensity values to produce a specific gradation curve for a particular image.

d. **True.** This may produce excessive shading across the image if not functioning correctly.

e. **False.** If the problem is related to a faulty image plate, then data processing techniques will not be able to improve the diagnostic quality of the final image if the artefact is significant.

11. a. **True.** Whatever the image acquisition technique (image plate or film), the presence of noise will reduce the ability to delineate areas of low contrast within the final image.

b. **False.** Noise is partly related to the efficiency of X-ray absorption by the image plate. A greater absorption efficiency will result in a better signal-to-noise ratio (SNR).

c. **False.** As with film-screen radiography, increasing the dose and the quantity of incident radiation will increase the SNR within the overall image.

d. **True.**

e. **True.** Neighbouring pixels with varying grey-scale values outside a particular range can be suppressed, resulting in an averaging of values and a smoothing out of the final image.

12. a. **True.** It is calculated as a ratio of the output signal-to-noise ratio (SNR) to the input SNR. The more efficient the system at recording this information, the greater the DQE.

b. **False.** The ratio is in the region of 0.4. A value of 1 implies that 100% of the X-ray information is recorded.

c. **False.** The opposite is true. Image plates of greater resolution will have a lower X-ray absorption efficiency due to a thinner phosphor layer and the absence of a light-reflective layer.

d. **True.** This allows laser-stimulated emission to occur simultaneously with summation of the output, increasing sensitivity.

e. **True.**

13. a. **True.**

b. **True.**

c. **False.** Different manufacturers of computed radiography systems will have different formulas for calculating the exposure index, and the relationship is not linear.

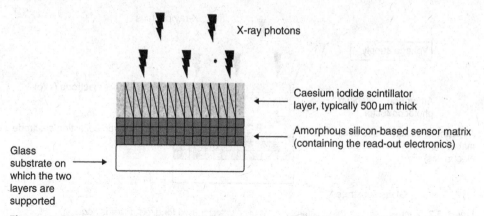

X-ray photons

Caesium iodide scintillator
layer, typically 500 μm thick

Amorphous silicon-based sensor matrix
(containing the read-out electronics)

Glass
substrate on
which the two
layers are
supported

Figure 5.1 Schematic view of the structure of a flat-plate detector used for indirect digital radiography.

   d. **True.**
   e. **False.** It is also related to the X-ray beam energy including filtration, the degree of scatter and the nature of the examination performed.

14. a. **False.** This is one of the main advantages of digital radiography.
   b. **True.** An amorphous silicon-based thin film transistor is used.
   c. **True.** This is typically caesium iodide.
   d. **False.** It is greater.
   e. **True.** Light from the scintillator is detected by a photodiode (one per pixel), which produces electrical charge. The charge is then stored within a capacitor. The thin-film transistor is then able to convert this charge into an electrical signal, which is then digitized into the image.

15. a. **True.**
   b. **True.** The DQE is 0.6 versus 0.4.
   c. **False.** The high speed relates to the amplification of the signal by the scintillator and the conversion gain by the photodiode.
   d. **True.**
   e. **True.**

16. a. **True.** The commonly used photoconductor is amorphous selenium.
   b. **True.** The photoconductor is usually bound to the amorphous silicon transistor array.
   c. **False.** Electrodes are placed across the photoconductor, which draws the released electrons and positively charged holes to the anode and cathode, respectively. The potential does not affect the absorption of the X-ray or the charge formed per photon.
   d. **False.** It is the positively charged holes that accumulate in the storage capacitors associated with each pixel. It is this charge that then forms the latent image by being digitized and transferred to the computer system.
   e. **False.** This is one of the main disadvantages.

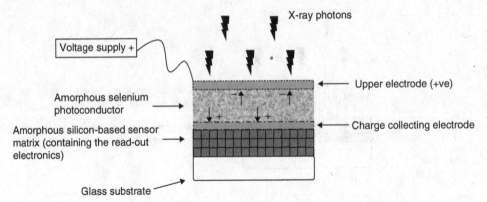

Figure 5.2 Schematic view of the structure of a flat-plate detector used for direct digital radiography.

17. a. **False.** The DQE of indirect conversion is greater.
   b. **True.** The K-edge of selenium is only 13 keV, which is less than the mean photon energy range used in general radiography. Much less of the incident X-ray beam will therefore be absorbed than with caesium iodide, which has K-edges of 36 keV and 33 keV.
   c. **False.** For the reasons mentioned in (b), the opposite is true. To achieve the same image quality, a higher patient dose is required with direct detectors.
   d. **True.** Again, this is related to differences in the DQE.
   e. **True.** Another measure of this is the modulation transfer factor, which is greater with direct than indirect conversion detectors. The differences relate to the direct transfer of electrical charge within the selenium, driven by the potential difference applied. With indirect detectors there is the possibility of light scatter within the scintillator, which increases unsharpness.

18. a. **True.**
   b. **True.** This relates to differences in the DQE.
   c. **False.** When using high-resolution image plates and a narrow laser beam for stimulated emission, a higher resolution is achievable with computed radiography.
   d. **False.** They are greater with digital radiography, as each radiographic machine needs its own detector, whereas with computed radiography the image plates may be used between existing machines. Costs may be saved later, however, as the patient throughput may be greater with digital radiography.
   e. **True.**

19. a. **False.** This refers to the variation in X-ray sensitivity, which may occur across the detector and be seen in the resultant image. This can be adjusted using gain calibration (so is not irreversible).
   b. **True.** This is compensated for by a process known as flat-field calibration. However, if there are a significant number of defective pixels, then image quality/accuracy may be compromised.
   c. **True.** If data are unprocessed, then the imaging display device may not be able to demonstrate the full range of intensities obtained. This is overcome by a process

known as auto-ranging, which processes the data to display only the most important part of the response range relevant to the particular examination performed.

d. **False.** It is an automatic process that is performed by software once details of the projection performed have been entered into the system, e.g. chest radiograph.

e. **False.**

20. a. **True.** This may be performed automatically based on the patient characteristics and the projection performed. It can also be manipulated directly by the operator.

b. **False.** It can improve contrast and brightness within the image.

c. **True.**

d. **True.** It improves the spatial resolution within the image.

e. **True.**

21. a. **False.** It is a scanning electron beam, which is directed at a phosphor, which produces the visible image. The intensity of the beam is varied, depending on the input of the signal.

b. **False.** After prolonged use, the image quality degrades, e.g. loss of contrast and problems with the phosphor.

c. **True.** The crystals vary in their degree of polarization when a voltage is placed across them. Each pixel can therefore be manipulated to vary the level of light transmission depending on the input of the signal to that pixel. The resultant image is a summation of all of the pixels.

d. **False.** A hardcopy may still be obtained using a laser hardware imager.

e. **False.**

22. a. **True.** With a typical digital matrix size of 3000 × 3000 and 2 bytes of data per pixel (at a minimum), then this is at least 18 Mb (matrix size × number of bytes) of data with a single image.

b. **False.** The reverse is true.

c. **True.**

d. **False.** Digital radiography uses larger matrix sizes.

e. **True.**

23. a. **True.** Although storage for hard-copy films is no longer required, it should be noted that data storage then becomes an issue.

b. **True.**

c. **True.** Reporting workstations usually have high-quality liquid crystal displays (LCDs), which are calibrated to the *Digital Imaging and Communications in Medicine* (DICOM) standard for that imaging modality. Within the hospital, PACS may be accessed from any PC connected to PACS via the hospital network. As images may be displayed on standard PC monitors, then reporting should be avoided at these workstations (in addition, the viewing environment may not be optimal).

d. **False.** They can, which is one of the main advantages of PACS over hard-copy images.

e. **True.**

24. a. **False.** There usually is more than one. A short-term archive exists for rapid accessing of images. A longer-term archive exists where the images are still available, but accessing them requires a longer period. This may be associated with data compression for storage.
   b. **True.**
   c. **True.** This allows the linking of patient administrative data along with the radiology information system (RIS).
   d. **True.** HL7 is a standard for the transfer of information regarding patient demographics, results and information from hospital systems.
   e. **False.** Although the costs associated with film and its storage are removed, the maintenance and upgrades to the PACS system (along with data storage) are continued, making the cost saving less evident.

25. a. **False.** DICOM is a standard for the handling and transmission of data associated with medical imaging. One of the benefits is to keep data for the image filed alongside information relating to the imaging modality and patient-identifying information.
   b. **True.**
   c. **False.** This service retrieves the scheduled worklist from the hospital information system (HIS) regarding examinations to be performed (hence reducing the need for repeated data entry) and may reduce data input errors.
   d. **True.**
   e. **True.**

26. a. **False.** It is still required.
   b. **False.** The Royal College of Radiologists (RCR) IT guidance (*Picture archiving and communication systems (PACS) and quality assurance*, 2008) recommends an ideal screen resolution of 3 megapixels and a screen size of at least 50 cm with at least a 10-bit grey scale.
   c. **True.** See the RCR IT guidance (*Picture archiving and communication systems (PACS) and quality assurance*, 2008).
   d. **True.**
   e. **True.** This is a standard look-up table against which different display devices should be calibrated to allow for varying device performances.

27. a. **True.** Film-screen radiography has a narrower dynamic range.
   b. **True.**
   c. **False.** Separation of these stages is the characteristic of digital radiography, which allows flexibility in the post-acquisition processing that may be performed.
   d. **False.**
   e. **True.**

28. a. **True.** Computed radiography has a dynamic range in the order of 10,000:1. Digital radiography has a dynamic range in the order of 1000:1 to 10,000:1. For both, the low end of the system is determined by noise. In digital radiography, the high end of the range is determined by the charge-holding capacity of the detector elements.

b. **False.** They are both affected by this. This is noise associated with the image receptor, which typically cannot be corrected for (so-called electronic noise).

c. **False.** This is related to an insufficient number of grey-scale values that can be demonstrated.

d. **True.**

e. **True.** Post-image acquisition analysis and processing can help with diagnosis of pathology.

29. a. **True.** This may be minimized by arranging the caesium iodide into narrow parallel columns, reducing the degree of reflection that may occur.

b. **False.** The larger the detector element, the more light or X-ray photons are detected by that element so that structures smaller than the detector size cannot be distinguished separately.

c. **False.** Increasing the thickness of the phosphor will increase the scattering of the laser light during image plate read-out.

d. **True.**

e. **True.**

30. a. **False.** Scatter of radiation occurs irrespective of the imaging system employed.

b. **True.** This is a type of internal source of noise (different to X-ray quantum noise) associated with the image receptor. Its contribution to the final image may be corrected for by using a control to obtain average values for the fixed system noise. This can then be used as a map to remove its contribution from subsequent images.

c. **True.** This may occur as a result of the manufacturing process. Compensation may occur by taking the average values from adjacent receptors and substituting these.

d. **False.** It can be used.

e. **True.** Due to decreased patient size, the image will have a different dynamic range than with adult patients and so digital enhancement needs to be varied to compensate for this.

Fluoroscopy and mammography – Questions

N. Sheikh-Bahaei

1. Regarding the intensifier in fluoroscopy:
   a. The chamber could be made of metal, e.g. aluminium, or of glass or ceramic
   b. It is filled with ionized gas
   c. There is a thin lead foil shielding the inner side of the chamber to prevent light from reaching the tube
   d. The anode is made of aluminium
   e. In fluoroscopy, γ is higher than in film-screen radiography

2. Regarding the input screen in fluoroscopy:
   a. Each absorbed X-ray photon gives rise to nearly 3000 light photons in the blue part of the spectrum
   b. The input phosphor is antimony caesium ($SbCs_3$)
   c. The input window is usually made of aluminium or titanium
   d. The phosphor thickness is 1–4 mm
   e. Only 60% of the incoming X-rays will be detected by the input phosphor

3. Regarding the output screen in the fluoroscopy:
   a. The output phosphor is silver-activated zinc cadmium sulphide (ZnCdS:Ag)
   b. The output phosphor emits green light
   c. The size of the output screen depends on the application
   d. The output phosphor is thicker than the input phosphor
   e. To reduce scatter in the output window, very thick glass can be used

4. Regarding image intensifiers in fluoroscopy:
   a. The diameter of the input screen is usually twice the diameter of the output screen
   b. The intensity of light produced in the input phosphor and the number of electrons produced by the photocathode are directly proportional to the intensity of the X-ray
   c. The sequence of interactions in an image intensifier tube is: X-ray $\rightarrow$ electrons $\rightarrow$ light $\rightarrow$ electrons
   d. Absorption of X-ray photons in the input screen window should be kept to a maximum
   e. X-ray scatter in the output window is a serious cause of contrast loss

5. Regarding gain in the image intensifier:
   a. The X-ray absorption efficiency of the input screen phosphor affects the gain of the image intensifier
   b. Flux gain means that a single light photon in the input phosphor causes multiple electrons in the photocathode

   c. The conversion factor provides a measure of image quality

   d. The conversion factor unit is $Cdm^2 (\mu Gy\ s^{-1})^{-1}$

   e. If the conversion factor for a 35 cm diameter input screen is 12, for a magnified field view with a 15 cm input screen the conversion factor would be 2.2

6. Regarding magnification in fluoroscopy:
   a. In the magnified mode, the focal point is closer to the output screen
   b. In magnification, both brightness and spatial resolution are increased
   c. Opening the iris aperture in front of the TV lens reduces the need to increase the dose rate in the magnified mode
   d. A change in voltage of the intermediate electrodes will magnify the image
   e. In the magnified view, both patient skin dose and effective dose increase in comparison with the full field of view without any collimation

7. Regarding the image distributor in fluoroscopy:
   a. To transfer the image from the intensifier to the TV system, a tandem lens pair is used
   b. As an automatic dose control, an electronic light sensor can be mounted between the two lenses to measure the brightness of the intensifier image
   c. The fluorographic camera is typically mounted parallel to the intensifier TV channel
   d. The output screen is in the focal plane of the primary collimating lens
   e. The physical structure mounted between the two lenses will affect the recorded image

8. Regarding the image recording device in fluoroscopy:
   a. In the TV camera tube, the light photons illuminate the heated cathode, which releases electrons
   b. In the TV camera tube, the scanning electron beam removes electrons from the inner surface of the target
   c. Each light photon absorbed in the charge-coupled device (CCD) gives rise to multiple electron–hole pairs
   d. CCD sensors have better resolution but less thermal and magnetic stability in comparison with a TV camera tube
   e. In CCD sensors, increasing the number of pixels improves the spatial resolution and negligible lag reduces the temporal unsharpness

9. Regarding the automatic brightness control (ABC):
   a. The ABC is made of three ionization chambers
   b. In new systems, the ABC measures the light intensity from the output screen
   c. In an anti-isowatt curve, both mA and kV increase with the an increase in radiological thickness
   d. An anti-isowatt curve is used in angiography
   e. The purpose of the ABC is to reduce the patient dose

10. Regarding the automatic brightness control (ABC) in fluoroscopy:
    a. In a high kV protocol, because the kV is at the maximum, the patient dose increases
    b. In a contrast study, the mA is kept near constant while the kV increases with radiological thickness
    c. Keeping the kV low and near constant maximizes the image quality but increases the patient dose

    d. A high kV mode is used in paediatric imaging

    e. In a contrast study with near-constant kV, the kV will never increase when the tube current reaches a certain level

11. Regarding automatic gain control:

    a. It means adjusting the image brightness seen in the monitor

    b. For automatic gain control, it is common to incorporate a mirror in the optics between two lenses

    c. It modifies the kV and mA according to the radiological thickness

    d. It increases the patient's dose relative to using automated brightness control when the radiological thickness is reduced

    e. It can be used to reduce an unnecessary dose to the patient

12. Regarding the dose rate in fluoroscopy:

    a. The detective quantum efficiency (DQE) is: (input screen signal/output screen brightness)^2

    b. The DQE is around 65% for a caesium iodide intensifier

    c. In fluoroscopy, the most critical limiting factor in dose rate is spatial resolution

    d. The dose rate at the input screen of the intensifier is commonly between 0.2 and 0.3 μGy s^{-1}

    e. With a change in the radiological thickness, the output signal will change significantly

13. Regarding the dose in fluoroscopy:

    a. In magnification, the brightness of the output screen increases in proportion to the reduction in area of the field of view

    b. The dose–area product (DAP) remains the same or is even reduced in the magnified view

    c. Camera gain is applied in the magnified view to reduce the input dose rate

    d. The entrance surface dose (ESD) and effective dose for each image are higher in the magnified view compared with the standard view without any collimation

    e. The ESD in a well-adjusted fluoroscopy system is around 100 mGy min^{-1}

14. In pulsed fluoroscopy:

    a. The pulse width is between 2 and 20 ms

    b. The dose rate falls approximately proportionally to the pulse rate

    c. Continuous fluoroscopy is often achieved using a pulse rate of around 30 pulses s^{-1}

    d. If there is no movement in the field of view, when the pulse rate falls below a certain level, it causes flickering of the image

    e. A higher pulse rate can produce a blurry image if there is movement in the field of view

15. In fluoroscopy:

    a. A grid-controlled tube is used to reduce the scatter in continuous fluoroscopy

    b. In a grid-controlled tube, there is a negative-voltage electrode between the anode and the cathode

    c. A digital spot image is the latest image of the fluorography on the TV monitor that can be saved

    d. A digital spot image is a low mA technique using a single pulse

    e. The dose for a digital spot image is between 0.1 and 0.5 mGy

16. In an analogue fluoroscopy system:

    a. The film in the cassette is linked to a selectable collimator so that multiple exposures can be made on a single film and multiple spot films can be saved on the same film

    b. Photospot images are about 30% of the size of what would be seen on the conventional spot film

    c. Photospot films have a short exposure time and they are noisy images

    d. For photospot images, a mirror between the output screen and the TV camera is used

    e. Synchronizing the pulse rate and frame rate is necessary to produce cine images

17. Regarding spatial resolution in fluoroscopy:

    a. Resolution is defined at the front face of the image intensifier

    b. Spatial resolution is limited by the spread of light in the input phosphor

    c. At the level of the output screen, the spatial resolution is 4–5 line pairs mm^{-1}

    d. On the display monitor, the spatial resolution is improved compared with the output screen

    e. In a magnified field of view, the spatial resolution in the display monitor is about 3 line pairs mm^{-1}

18. Regarding image quality in fluoroscopy:

    a. The signal-to-noise ratio (SNR) will improve by increasing the image intensification or camera gain

    b. The veiling glare is only from the light scattering in the output window and is not affected by scattering of the X-rays in the input screen

    c. Veiling glare means a blurry line surrounding the image

    d. Vignetting means the periphery of the image is brighter than the centre

    e. The larger the intensifier, the greater the veiling effect

19. Regarding factors affecting the image:

    a. Curvature of the output screen causes a pin cushion effect

    b. S-type distortion is caused by the magnetic field influencing the path of electrons

    c. Images in intensifiers are magnified towards the centre

    d. The vignetting effect is reduced by curving the input screen

    e. Less electron focusing at the periphery causes less distortion at the peripheral parts of the image

20. Regarding the testing of image quality:

    a. To check the spatial resolution of the system, a high kV method is used

    b. The grid for spatial resolution testing is positioned parallel to the matrix

    c. For contrast resolution, a low-contrast test object is used

    d. The test object for contrast resolution contains circular inserts of high atomic number

    e. The Leeds test object is used for contrast resolution testing

21. Regarding digital subtraction angiography (DSA):
    a. It is a high-dose technique with a lower dose of contrast medium
    b. Misregistration is more prominent at the boundaries between low-contrast details
    c. Pixel shifting can be done for each movement in the field of view
    d. The signals of the contrast and mask images are converted into their logarithms prior to subtraction because of the exponential nature of the attenuation
    e. Taking several mask and contrast images, with later subtraction according to the table position, will need less examination time but more contrast medium

22. Regarding dual-energy subtraction:
    a. A high kV image displays a high contrast between bone and soft tissues
    b. At low kV, the image contrast is influenced by tissue density rather than atomic number
    c. Subtraction of the low kV from the high kV image improves the soft tissue contrast
    d. Subtraction of the high kV from the low kV image displays bony details
    e. This technique involves taking three images: mask, low kV and high kV in rapid succession

23. Regarding flat-plate detectors:
    a. Caesium iodide is used as the scintillator
    b. They have the same detective quantum efficiency (DQE) as a conventional image intensifier
    c. They have the same dynamic range as a conventional image intensifier
    d. In a magnified field of view, the spatial resolution is increased
    e. Both contrast resolution and distortion are less in comparison with a conventional image intensifier

24. In mammography:
    a. A low tube potential is needed because of the small irradiated tissue
    b. The film has a smaller latitude compared with general radiography
    c. The screen is made of caesium iodide
    d. Single-sided emulsion is used on the inner side of the film
    e. The principal interaction is the photoelectric effect with L-shell electrons

25. Regarding targets and filters in mammography:
    a. The Rh–Mo target–filter combination is used for thicker breast tissue
    b. Using a Rh filter with a Mo target increases the mean and peak photon energy of the spectrum compared with Mo–Mo
    c. Rh produces a characteristic radiation slightly lower than Mo
    d. The combination of W–Rh has the best contrast
    e. In the Mo–Mo combination, the dose is higher than in other combinations

26. Regarding mammography units:
    a. Spatial resolution is 8–10 line pairs mm^{-1}
    b. The anode is on the chest wall side
    c. The focal spot size for the magnified view is 0.3 mm
    d. The axial ray is directed to the centre of the X-ray field
    e. The focus-to-film distance (FFD) is fixed in mammography

27. Regarding image quality in mammography:
    a. Compression reduces movement unsharpness but has no effect on geometrical unsharpness
    b. A magnified view increases unsharpness
    c. A linear moving grid is generally used in mammography to reject scatter in more than one direction
    d. The mammography unit is designed to overcome the anode heel effect
    e. A typical compression force is 100–150 N

28. Regarding quality assurance in mammography:
    a. Small-field digital tests need to be carried out on a daily basis
    b. Testing the automatic exposure control (AEC) consistency with thickness variation is performed daily
    c. The function of the compression device should be checked monthly
    d. kV accuracy can be checked monthly
    e. Image quality should be checked weekly

29. Regarding the dose and dose measurement in mammography:
    a. The dose and breast thickness are directly proportional
    b. In a single-sided screen, the resolution is better but a higher dose is required
    c. Automatic exposure control (AEC) terminates the exposure after a fixed dose to the detector
    d. By varying kV, a greater dose saving can be made for the same loss in contrast, in comparison with changing the target–filter combination
    e. The entrance surface dose (ESD) is proportional to tube kV^2

30. Which of the following are typical features of a mammography set?
    a. The automatic exposure control (AEC) detector is placed behind the cassette
    b. The anode does not rotate
    c. Multiple targets and filters are used
    d. A variable field size is used
    e. A small-field digital system is used for stereo localization

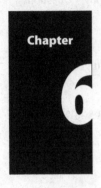

Fluoroscopy and mammography – Answers

1. a. **True**. It is an evacuated chamber made of glass, ceramic or metal such as aluminium.
   b. **False**. It is an evacuated glass, ceramic or metal chamber.
   c. **False**. It is surrounded by metal housing, preventing light from reaching the tube and shielding it from the effect of the magnetic field.
   d. **True**. The inner surface of the output screen is coated with a very thin layer of aluminium, which acts as the anode.
   e. **False**. There is a direct relationship between the brightness displayed on the output screen and the intensity of the X-ray photons falling on the input phosphor: doubling the X-ray exposure doubles the light output ($\gamma = 1$), in contrast to film-screen radiography ($\gamma = 2$–3).

2. a. **True**.
   b. **False**. It is caesium iodide.
   c. **True**. The input window provides protection for the sensitive input components of the tube and maintains the vacuum. The input window is usually fabricated from a low-atomic-number metal, for example, aluminium ($Z = 13$) or titanium ($Z = 22$) foil. Therefore, the X-ray beam can enter the image intensifier with minimum attenuation. It also provides mechanical rigidity and maintains the vacuum.
   d. **False**. The phosphor thickness is 0.1–0.4 mm.
   e. **True**.

3. a. **True**.
   b. **True**.
   c. **False**. The input screen size is 150–400 mm in diameter and its size depends on the application: smaller for orthopaedic applications and largest for angiography and interventional radiology. The output screen size does not change according to application.
   d. **False**. The output phosphor is thinner than the input phosphor.
   e. **True**. Scatter of light, or halation, in the output window can seriously degrade the contrast of the output image. Anti-halation techniques typically include the use of smoked glass, special optical coatings, very thick glass or a fibre-optic bundle.

4. a. **False**. The input screen diameter is ten times that of the output screen.
   b. **True**.
   c. **False**. It is X-ray → light → electrons → light
   d. **False**. see Q2, answer c.
   e. **False**. Scatter of light in the output window affects the contrast.

5. a. **False.** Gain is affected by minification, and flux gain; the efficiency of the input screen does not affect the gain.
    b. **False.** Flux gain means a single light photon produced in the input phosphor causes a single electron in the photocathode but multiple photons in the output screen.
    c. **False.** The conversion factor is a useful measure of gain but does not provide a measure of image quality.
    d. **False.** It is Cd m^{-2} (μGy s^{-1})$^{-1}$.
    e. **True.** $12 \times (15/35)^2 = 2.2$.

6. a. **False.** It is closer to the input screen.
    b. **False.** In the magnified mode, the spatial resolution is higher but the gain (brightness) is less.
    c. **True.** A circular iris aperture of adjustable diameter is normally used to calibrate the light intensity illuminating the image recording device. The iris aperture is also used to compensate (at least in part) for the fall in gain when a magnified field is selected. Opening the iris aperture reduces the need to increase the dose rate to compensate for such a fall in gain.
    d. **True.**
    e. **False.** Magnification reduces the brightness on the output screen, and to restore the brightness the exposure factors increase, thus increasing the patient's skin dose. However, because the surface area is reduced, the effective dose would be less in comparison with a full field of view without collimation.

7. a. **True.** An optical distributor is a light-tight housing that contains the optical components required to transfer the image from the output screen to the TV sensor. Image transfer takes place via a so-called tandem lens pair. The tandem lens pair comprises two optics, one associated with the intensifier and the other with the TV sensor (Fig.6.1).
    b. **True.** An electronic light sensor is mounted between the two lenses to measure the brightness of the intensifier image and can be used as a real-time feedback signal for an automatic dose (rate) control system. These are used to automatically adjust the intensifier input dose rate to take account of differences in X-ray transmission through different body sections of the patient and for patients of different sizes.
    c. **False.** When a fluorographic camera is implemented, it is typically mounted at a right angle to the intensifier TV channel.
    d. **True.** The output screen lies in the focal plane of the primary collimating lens and therefore the image is effectively focused an infinite distance away (Fig.6.1).
    e. **False.** The image is completely out of focus for any optical plane in the space between the two lenses. This design brings the added benefit that physical structures can be mounted between the two lens and they will not appear in the recorded image (Fig.6.1).

8. a. **False.** The image recording device first used in intensifier TV fluoroscopy was the TV camera tube. This comprises a cylindrical evacuated glass tube with a light-sensitive target in the front face, which is illuminated by light photons from the output screen of the intensifier, and a heated cathode as a high-resolution electron source mounted at the opposite end of the tube (Fig.6.2).

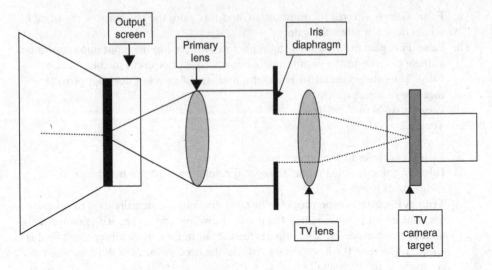

Figure 6.1 Diagram of a TV fluoroscopy channel tandem lens pair.

b. **False.** The scanning electron beam is scanned over the target and deposits electrons on the surface, building up a uniform charge density (Fig.6.2).

c. **False.** Each light photon (from the intensifier output) absorbed in the silicon substrate of the CCD gives rise to an electron–hole pair. The quantity of electronic charge that accumulates at each pixel is directly proportional to the intensity of the incident light and the frame integration time.

d. **False.** The technological benefits of CCD sensors include:
- Small, inexpensive and compact with low power consumption
- Self-scanning image readout (no large electromagnetic deflection coils required)
- Negligible lag (less temporal unsharpness)
- Resilience against burned-in signals at high-intensity lights
- Geometrical precision and spatial uniformity
- Excellent thermal, electrical and magnetic stability
- Excellent serviceability and long life-time
- Compatibility with digital X-ray imaging modalities

e. **True.** Spatial resolution can be improved by increasing the number of pixels in the array.

9. a. **False.** The automatic exposure control (AEC) is usually made of three ionization chambers in diagnostic radiology.

b. **False.** In modern systems, it is usual to take the camera signal to provide information for the ABC.

c. **True.**

d. **False.** In angiography, the system holds the tube potential between 60 and 65 kV and the mA increases with radiological thickness.

e. **False.** Some protocols are designed to maximize the image quality but at the cost of an increased dose because of low kV.

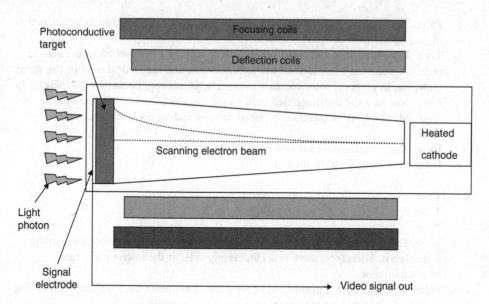

Figure 6.2 Diagram of a tube TV camera.

10. a. **False.** This technique minimizes the dose at the cost of image quality; it is suitable for paediatrics.
    b. **False.** The kV is held between 60 and 65, and with increased radiological thickness the mA is increased.
    c. **True.**
    d. **True.**
    e. **False.** For a radiological thickness that would need higher tube currents, the system increases the kV while reducing the mA to ensure that the maximum power is not exceeded.

11. a. **True.**
    b. **False.** Automatic gain control is achieved by adjusting the sensitivity (gain) of the TV system itself.
    c. **False.** mA and kV are not altered as radiological thickness changes.
    d. **True.**
    e. **True.** In fluoroscopy, the automatic gain control can reduce the patient's dose at the cost of increased image noise.

12. a. **False.** DQE is: (output brightness/input signal)^2.
    b. **True.**
    c. **False.** Noise is the main limiting factor.
    d. **True.**
    e. **False.** As the thickness changes, kV and mA are adjusted to keep the output brightness or camera signal at a nearly constant level with relatively small variations to input dose rate.

13. a. **False.** The brightness of the output image is decreased in proportion to the reduction in area of the field of view.
   b. **True.** The input dose rate must be increased in inverse proportion to the area in order to retain the same level of image brightness, and the DAP should be the same. However, in practice, some increase in camera gain is applied so that the increase in input dose rate for the magnified field of view is less than would otherwise be required. The DAP is therefore reduced to some extent on magnification.
   c. **True.**
   d. **False.** The effective dose for one image does not increase.
   e. **False.** It is around 10–30 mGy min^{-1}.

14. a. **True.**
   b. **True.**
   c. **True.**
   d. **False.** Each successive image is retained on the display until the following image is displayed. Therefore, there is no flickering, even at the lowest pulse rate, in a static scene.
   e. **False.** With movement in the field of view, the lower pulse rates will display blurring or lag, which may be unacceptable for a particular examination.

15. a. **False.** Grid-controlled tubes are used in pulsed-mode fluoroscopy.
   b. **True.** In a grid-controlled tube, there is an electrode between the cathode and anode with a negative voltage relative to the cathode of approximately 2 kV.
   c. **False.** A fluoro-grab image is the latest frame displayed on the TV monitor that can be stored permanently as a record or for subsequent reporting.
   d. **False.** A digital spot image is a single-shot image taken with a single pulse of radiation at a high mA to produce a low-noise image.
   e. **False.** It is between 0.1 and 5 µGy.

16. a. **True.** In analogue systems, recording was principally done by film-screen radiography; the cassette with the film in place was automatically driven into the position in front of the intensifier and the exposure made, with a time delay between initiation and exposure of <1 s. The film and cassette are linked to a selectable collimator so that multiple exposures can be made on a single film, which is referred to as a spot film.
   b. **True.** An alternative method of taking spot films was to use a camera attached to the image intensifier using a mirror introduced between the output screen and the TV camera, then take a picture of the image on the output screen of the intensifier. The film size was 105 mm, about 30% of the size of what would be seen on the conventional spot film. These films are referred to as photospot images.
   c. **False.** Photospot films have a short exposure time and increased mA, resulting in reduced noise.
   d. **True.**
   e. **True.** By synchronizing the pulse rate and frame rate, cine recordings can be made.

17. a. **True.**
   b. **False.** Spatial resolution is limited by the spread of light in the output phosphor.
   c. **True.**

  d. **False.** The resolution on the monitor is more limited because of the degradation in TV. The theoretical spatial resolution is 1.7 line pairs mm^{-1}.
  e. **True.**

18. a. **False.** For an image intensifier, quantum sink corresponds to the photons absorbed in the input screen. Increasing the image intensifier or camera gain will not improve the SNR.
  b. **False.** Veiling glare is mainly from light scattering in the output window but also by X-rays and light scattering in the input phosphor and electron scattering in the tube itself.
  c. **False.** It means dark regions in the image appearing lighter because of the surrounding light areas.
  d. **False.** It means that the central area of the image is brighter than the periphery.
  e. **True.**

19. a. **False.** Curvature of the input screen is responsible for the pin cushion effect.
  b. **True.**
  c. **False.** They are magnified towards the edges; this is called the pin cushion effect.
  d. **True.**
  e. **False.** Electrons are less focused at the periphery causing increased brightness and resolution in the centre and less distortion in the centre; these effects are more pronounced in a larger intensifier.

20. a. **False.** A low kV method is used to reduce scatter and maximize contrast.
  b. **False.** The grid is generally angled at 45° with respect to the matrix in order to avoid interference artefacts on the displayed image.
  c. **True.**
  d. **True.** Contrast resolution is tested with a low-contrast test object, such as a Leeds test object, comprising a flat disc 6 mm thick and 200–300 mm in diameter containing circular inserts of high-atomic-number material that produce varying levels of contrast.
  e. **True.**

21. a. **True.**
  b. **False.** Misregistration is caused by movement, particularly at the boundaries between high-contrast details, e.g. bone edges.
  c. **False.** Pixel shifting can be done over the full area of the image and does not allow for differential movement within the field of view.
  d. **True.**
  e. **False.** Most DSA allows acquisition of several mask and contrast images along the full length by table movement. The table position is recorded for each contrast image. The system will subtract the appropriate mask image according to the table position. The advantages of this method are less contrast medium and less time required for examination.

22. a. **False.** A low kV image displays a high contrast between bone and soft tissues.
  b. **False.** At high kV, the contrast of bone is significantly reduced, and image contrast is influenced by tissue density rather than atomic number.
  c. **True.**

  d. **True.**
  e. **False.** No mask image is needed.

23. a. **True.**
  b. **True.** The DQE for these detectors is comparable with an image intensifier (about 65%).
  c. **False.** The principal advantages of these detectors are increased dynamic range and improved spatial resolution.
  d. **False.** The spatial resolution when using a flat-plate detector does not improve with magnification.
  e. **False.** The contrast resolution is better and distortion is less.

24. a. **False.** A low tube potential is needed to maximize the low-contrast subject.
  b. **True.** In mammography, there is not much difference between the different tissues imaged. Therefore, mammography film has a small latitude, i.e. the range of exposure needed to cover the grey scale is reduced, so that a small change in exposure gives an enhanced change in blackening of the film. This means that mammography film has a very steep linear part of the sensitometric curve.
  c. **False.** It is made of rare earth materials.
  d. **False.** Single-sided emulsion is used on the distal side of the film.
  e. **True.**

25. a. **False.** The combination of Rh-Mo is not used, because the effect of the filter would be to attenuate the Rh characteristic radiation with energy that is just greater than the K-edge of Mo.
  b. **False.** Use of a Mo–Rh combination increases the mean energy of the spectrum, because it will transmit Bremsstrahlung photons in the energy range just below 23.2 keV, thus increasing the beam penetration, but peak photon energy is determined by the tube potential and the target material does not affect this.
  c. **False.** The characteristic radiation of Rh is 23.2 keV and Mo is 20 keV.
  d. **False.** Contrast in different target–filter combinations decreases as follows: Mo–Mo > Mo–Rh > Rh–Rh > W–Rh.
  e. **True.** The dose in different target–filter combinations decreases as follows: Mo–Mo > Mo–Rh > Rh–Rh > W–Rh.

26. a. **False.** Spatial resolution is 15 line pairs mm^{-1} or above.
  b. **False.** The cathode is on the chest wall side.
  c. **False.** For the magnified view, the smaller focal spot size is used, which is 0.1–0.15 mm. The larger one (0.4 mm) is for the standard view.
  d. **False.** The tube is angled so that the axial ray is at the chest wall edge; this helps to produce films with a more uniform density.
  e. **True.** Unlike general X-ray equipment, the distance between the tube head and the film cannot usually be varied. This is because the set is designed for a single examination and the focus-to-film distance used is considered the optimum. The normal FFD is 65 or 66 cm.

27. a. **False.** Compression reduces both geometrical and movement unsharpness, as well as scatter.
  b. **True.**

c. **False.** In mammography, moving grids are used for all normal contact images. The grids are generally linear, i.e. they reject scatter in one direction and move from side to side during the exposure, so that they are not seen on the images. Sometimes the exposure stops momentarily when the grid reaches one end of its path to prevent its image appearing on the film. If the exposure times are very short or if the grid speed is not set correctly, then grid lines can sometimes be seen on the image.

d. **False.** The radiation across the X-ray beam is not uniform due to the anode heel effect. However, in mammography what we are imaging is not of uniform thickness. A breast is more like a cone in shape. If a uniform X-ray beam were applied to a breast, the resultant density of the film would vary across the breast, being highest where the breast is thinnest (nipple edge) and lowest where the breast is thickest (chest wall edge). We want a uniform film density. To help achieve this we make use of the anode heel effect. In general radiography, the highest intensity part of the X-ray beam is in the centre of the field. In mammography, we want the highest intensity part of the beam to coincide with the thickest part of the breast, i.e. the chest wall edge. To achieve this, the tube is angled and collimated.

e. **True.** The compression paddle can be moved up and down by a powered motor. During an examination, the compression paddle will slowly be brought down on to the breast. This compresses the breast to make it thinner. The maximum force applied should be no greater than 200 N (equivalent to an approximately 20 kg weight). Standard compression forces are normally between 100 and 150 N.

28. a. **True.** These are the main tests that might be performed on a daily basis:
   - Automatic exposure control (AEC) consistency
   - Film processor sensitometry
   - Small-field digital tests
   - Cassette cleaning
   - Inspection of breast support table and associated equipment

   b. **False.** These are the main tests that might be performed weekly:
   - AEC consistency with thickness variation
   - Image quality
   - Stereotactic localizing device

   c. **True.** These are the main tests that might be performed monthly:
   - Mechanical safety and function of the compression device
   - Densitometer calibration

   d. **False.** The following should be tested every 6 months:
   - kV accuracy
   - X-ray output
   - Filtration and half-value layer (HVL)
   - Focal spot size

   e. **True.**

29. a. **False.** For larger breasts, the doses are much higher than for average breasts, as there is a greater thickness of material for the radiation to penetrate and so more is absorbed. Also, loss of reciprocity in the film means even larger doses are needed to achieve the right film density. However, the dose is not linear and rises more steeply after about 6 cm (Fig.6.3).

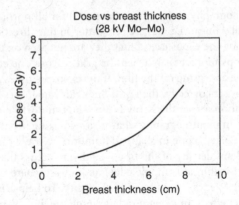

Figure 6.3 Graph showing the relationship between dose and breast thickness.

b. **True.** A back screen means that, as most interactions still take place at the edge of the screen nearest to the radiation source, the film is nearer the interaction, i.e. light source, and the light does not spread out as much, giving a better resolution.
By using single-sided film, the emulsion is in direct contact with the screen and the resolution is therefore as good as possible. However, use of a single screen and single-sided emulsion means than a higher dose is required than if doubled-sided film with two screens were used.

c. **False.** Due to beam hardening, the amount of radiation dose reaching the detector varies with breast thickness and composition. If the AEC worked by detecting a fixed dose, film density would vary with breast variation.

d. **False.** By varying the kV, you can reduce the dose and exposure time. However, by changing the target–filter combination, a greater dose saving can be made for the same loss in contrast, or a lower loss in contrast can be achieved for the same dose decrease.

e. **False.** Increasing the kV does increase the output of the X-ray tube and the ESD, but output at mammographic energies is roughly proportional to kV^3. In general radiography, output is approximately proportional to kV^2.

30. a. **True.** In general radiography, the AEC detector is normally placed between the patient and the film. However, if this were the case in mammography, the AEC device would be visible on the images and for this reason, the AEC detector is placed behind the cassette.

b. **False.** If the anode did not rotate, it would not cope with being heated.

c. **True.**

d. **False.** Mammographic equipment has fixed field sizes, normally 18 × 24 cm and 24 × 30 cm.

e. **True.** Small-field digital technology is now the standard method used for stereo localization. When a small-field digital system is used for stereo localization, the image is normally available within 30 s of the exposure and no film handling is required. This significantly reduces the procedure time, which means that movement of the patient is a much smaller issue. It also reduces the total time for the procedure.

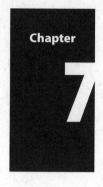

Nuclear medicine – Questions

S. Ilyas

1. Which of the following are true with regard to isotopes of a given element?
   a. They have the same number of nucleons
   b. They have the same atomic mass
   c. They differ in densities
   d. They have the same number of protons but a different number of electrons
   e. They have the same position on the periodic table

2. Which of the following statements are correct, when referring to an atom?
   a. The valence shell is responsible for radioactivity
   b. Radioactivity results from an imbalance in the number of protons and electrons
   c. All atoms have an equal number of protons and neutrons
   d. Neutrons have a negative charge
   e. Radon contributes to our background radiation

3. The production of radionuclides can involve:
   a. The addition of a neutron into a stable nucleus
   b. Capturing a negative electron from the K-shell (electron capture)
   c. Addition of a proton into the nucleus using a nuclear reactor
   d. The use of a cyclotron
   e. Removal of electrons from the inner shell

4. Concerning radionuclide production:
   a. Radionuclides used in medicine are generally found naturally
   b. In a cyclotron, protons are forced into the nucleus
   c. In a nuclear reactor, the addition of a neutron into the nucleus results in an increase in atomic number
   d. Radionuclides produced in a cyclotron can be separated from the stable (carrier) element
   e. Radionuclides produced in a nuclear reactor by neutron capture alone can be separated from the stable (carrier) element

5. Regarding radioactive decay:
   a. K-electron capture is a type of radioactive decay process
   b. It is a stochastic process
   c. It can occur following an increase in electron numbers
   d. It results in absorption of energy from the surrounding atoms
   e. It always results in a stable daughter nucleus

6. Which of the following are correct with regard to beta-negative (β^-) decay?
   a. It involves the ejection of a positron (positive electron)
   b. It results in increased atomic number
   c. It results in increased atomic mass
   d. It results in a daughter nucleus with a high energy state
   e. It occurs in a neutron-deficient radionuclide

7. Concerning the properties of nuclear isomers:
   a. They have different atomic numbers
   b. They have the same atomic mass
   c. They have the same half-life
   d. They have different energy states
   e. The metastable isomer is formed following the release of the gamma ray

8. Which of the following are correct with regard to beta-positive (β^+) decay?
   a. It occurs in a radionuclide with a neutron excess
   b. Radionuclides become stable by a neutron changing to a proton
   c. It results in reduced atomic number
   d. It results in increased atomic mass
   e. It results in ejection of a positron

9. Following electron capture:
   a. The number of protons increases
   b. The atom is negatively charged
   c. The atomic mass stays the same
   d. The atomic number is reduced
   e. Bremsstrahlung radiation is released

10. Which of the following are true regarding gamma rays?
    a. They are released following the interaction of electrons with a tungsten target
    b. They have a mass
    c. They form a line spectrum, representing energy levels that are specific to the nuclide that emits them
    d. They have a frequency proportional to their energy
    e. They can be absorbed within the emitting atom

11. Regarding beta radiation:
    a. It is made up of photons
    b. It is emitted with a continuous spectrum of energy
    c. The maximum energy of the electron is dependent on the radionuclide material
    d. The distance travelled by a beta particle is inversely proportional to the density of the material through which it is travelling
    e. Beta rays travel in a straight line

12. The following are true regarding beta particles and their interactions:
    a. Both electrons and positrons have a mass
    b. Beta particles result in a trail of ionized atoms

c. The collision of two positrons results in complete annihilation of the two particles

d. Positron annihilation results in the release of gamma photons

e. Beta particles increase the temperature of the surrounding tissue

13. Which of the following are true regarding radioactive decay?
   a. The unit of radioactive decay is the becquerel (Bq)
   b. Beta-particle emitters used in nuclear medicine can only be produced in a nuclear reactor
   c. Radioactive decay rate is measured by absorbed energy (kg of tissue)$^{-1}$ min^{-1}
   d. The lower the number of radioactive atoms in a sample, the greater the count rate
   e. A radionuclide will always undergo radioactive decay within the known half-life of the isotope

14. Which of the following are true regarding radioactivity?
   a. The radioactivity decay of a radionuclide decreases by equal fractions (%) in equal intervals of time
   b. The rate of decay (activity of the radioactive material) is proportional to the count rate
   c. The count rate is always less than the radioactive decay rate
   d. The radioactive sample eventually decays completely, resulting in no activity
   e. The lower the number of radioactive atoms in a sample, the lower the rate of decay

15. Regarding the half-life of a radionuclide:
   a. It allows an estimation of how long it will take for a given sample to decay to half its activity
   b. The time taken for a given quantity to decay to half its activity reduces as the sample gets smaller
   c. Isotopes with a short half-life are considered more radioactive than those with longer half-lives
   d. Radionuclides produced in a cyclotron are known to have shorter half-lives than those produced in a generator
   e. Tc-99m has a half-life of about 6 h

16. Which of the following are true regarding the biological half-life of a radiopharmaceutical?
   a. It is dependent on the rate of radioactive decay of the radiopharmaceutical within the body
   b. It may increase as a result of organ failure
   c. It is used to calculate the effective half-life
   d. It is shorter than the effective half-life
   e. It is the same for a given radiopharmaceutical in every individual

17. Which of the following are true regarding the physical half-life of a radiopharmaceutical?
   a. It is the rate at which a radiopharmaceutical agent is physically eliminated from the body
   b. Body temperature must be taken into consideration when estimating the physical half-life of a radiopharmaceutical within a patient's body

c. It is used to calculate how much radiopharmaceutical agent to prepare depending on its time of use

d. It differs according to the pharmaceutical agent used

e. It increases when placed in an acidic solution

18. Regarding the effective half-life of a radionuclide:
    a. It takes into account the biological and physical half-lives
    b. It decreases as a result of renal failure
    c. The dose received by an organ is proportional to the effective half-life
    d. It differs among individuals for a given radiopharmaceutical
    e. It is generally increased in patients with liver failure

19. Desirable properties of a radionuclide for imaging include:
    a. High levels of cross-reactivity with blood proteins
    b. A half-life measured in hours, not minutes or days
    c. It decays to a stable daughter
    d. Low activity per unit volume
    e. Emission of beta particles

20. Which of the following are desirable properties of gamma rays produced by radionuclides for imaging?
    a. The energy of the photon should be more than 100 keV
    b. Emission of polyenergetic gamma rays
    c. High energy
    d. Low energy
    e. Emission of pure gamma rays

21. Which of the following are desirable properties of a pharmaceutical agent for imaging?
    a. It easily accumulates in all tissues
    b. It has a long biological half-life
    c. It should be stable after labelling with a radionuclide
    d. It emits gamma rays
    e. It has a high affinity for the target organ or tissue

22. Concerning Tc-99m:
    a. It is the daughter nucleus of Mo-99 and is produced following the emission of gamma rays
    b. Tc-99m and Tc-99 differ in their half-lives
    c. It emits gamma rays with 140 keV
    d. Pertechnetate (TcO_4^-) is used in imaging to localize Meckel's diverticulum
    e. It emits beta particles

23. Which of the following are true regarding the sensitivity of collimators?
    a. It is a measure of the fraction of total gamma rays falling on the collimator that pass through the holes to the crystal
    b. Increasing the number of holes increases the sensitivity
    c. Increasing the sensitivity reduces the patient dose

   d. Narrower holes result in increased sensitivity
   e. Longer holes reduce sensitivity

24. Regarding collimators:
   a. For parallel hole collimators, the field of view and sensitivity do not change with distance
   b. Sensitivity is inversely proportional to the spatial resolution
   c. Convergent collimators result in an inverted image
   d. Divergent collimators allow the use of a small crystal to image a large field of view
   e. Spatial resolution improves by reducing the distance from the patient

25. Which of the following concerning gamma cameras are true?
   a. The primary purpose of the collimator is to filter out low-energy gamma rays
   b. Photomultipliers convert light into photoelectrons
   c. The pulse height analyser reduces noise
   d. Low-energy gamma rays result from photoelectric absorption in the crystal and patient
   e. Spatial resolution can be improved by using collimators with wider holes

26. Regarding the crystal used in gamma cameras:
   a. It is usually made of NaI due to its robust qualities
   b. It absorbs gamma rays mainly by photoelectric absorption
   c. The absorption of a single gamma proton results in the production of a single light photon
   d. Using a thicker crystal improves intrinsic resolution
   e. A crack in the crystal results in a linear defect on a uniform background

27. Which of the following are true regarding spatial resolution?
   a. Intrinsic resolution refers to resolution from the camera and collimator
   b. The addition of a collimator decreases intrinsic resolution further
   c. The larger the patient, the worse the spatial resolution
   d. Spatial resolution can be tested using a bar test pattern
   e. Spatial resolution can be tested by imaging a line source

28. Concerning the sensitivity of gamma cameras (system sensitivity):
   a. It is a function of both intrinsic and collimator efficiency
   b. At high keV, the intrinsic sensitivity is almost 100%
   c. Using a thicker crystal increases sensitivity
   d. It is measured using a bar test
   e. It is expressed as total counts per second per megabecquerel of activity (cps MBq^{-1})

29. Single-photon emission tomography (SPECT) is different to conventional gamma imaging in which of the following ways?
   a. It results in improved target-to-background ratios
   b. It results in improved spatial resolution
   c. It uses a rotating gamma camera
   d. It results in a higher number of counts for a given acquisition time
   e. It results in images that can be reconstructed to form 3D images

30. Which of the following are true with regard to positron emission tomography (PET)?
    a. It detects single gamma rays produced following the collision of a positron with a negative beta particle
    b. The radionuclides used in PET are normally produced in a cyclotron
    c. It results in lower noise levels than conventional gamma imaging
    d. It provides detailed anatomical information
    e. Scintillation detectors are usually made of NaI

Nuclear medicine – Answers

1. a. **False.** Nucleon is a collective term for neutrons and protons. Isotopes of the same element have the same number of protons but a different number of neutrons.
   b. **False.** Atomic mass is equal to the number of protons and neutrons in a nucleus. Isotopes differ in the number of neutrons and therefore have different atomic mass numbers.
   c. **True.** Isotopes differ in many of their physical properties including their densities.
   d. **False.** The number of orbiting electrons (negative charge) is equal to the number of protons (positive charge).
   e. **True.** Elements are positioned in the periodic table according to their atomic number (number of protons), which remains the same for isotopes of the same element.

2. a. **False.** The valence shell is the outer electron shell and influences the chemical and thermal properties of an atom. Radioactivity involves the nucleus.
   b. **False.** Radioactivity occurs as a result of unstable nuclei (radionuclide) that have an excess or deficit of neutrons.
   c. **False.** For example, hydrogen has one proton only and no neutrons.
   d. **False.** Neutrons have no charge. Protons have a positive charge and electrons have a negative charge.
   e. **True.** Radon is an example of a naturally occurring radionuclide.

3. a. **True.** This is one of the methods by which radionuclides are produced. The process takes place in a nuclear reactor.
   b. **False.** Electron capture is a form of radioactive decay.
   c. **False.** The forceful addition of a proton into the nucleus causing the ejection of a neutron is also one of the methods by which radionuclides are produced. However, this process takes place in a cyclotron, which accelerates charged particles, e.g. protons, onto the target material.
   d. **True.**
   e. **False.** Radioactivity involves the nucleus.

4. a. **False.** Radionuclides used in medicine are produced artificially.
   b. **True.** A cyclotron accelerates protons (and other charged particles) onto the target material, resulting in the addition of the proton into the nucleus, causing a neutron to be ejected.
   c. **False.** Atomic number is equal to the number of protons, which is unchanged in this particular process unless the addition of a neutron causes nuclear instability and the expulsion of a proton, in which case the atomic number will decrease.

d. **True.** Radionuclides produced in a cyclotron can be separated from their carrier as they have different atomic numbers and hence different chemical properties.

e. **False.** Radionuclides produced in a nuclear reactor by neutron capture cannot be separated from the stable compound (carrier) as they have the same atomic number and hence the same chemical properties.

5. a. **True.** Neutron deficient radionuclides increase their number of neutrons relative to protons by capturing an electron from the K-shell.

b. **True.**

c. **False.** Radioactive decay occurs due to the nuclei being unstable as a result of either an excess or a deficiency in the number of neutrons or protons.

d. **False.** Radioactive decay is not an energy-dependent process and occurs independently.

e. **False.** Although radioactive decay can result in a stable daughter nucleus, a metastable or unstable daughter nucleus may also be formed.

6. a. **False.** Radionuclides lose energy and become stable in beta decay by a neutron changing to a proton plus an electron. The electron is ejected from the nucleus with high energy and is referred to as a negative beta particle.

b. **True.** There is an increase in the number of protons (atomic number).

c. **False.**

d. **True.** The daughter nucleus is produced with excess energy and loses this as gamma photons.

e. **False.** Beta-negative (β^-) decay occurs in a radionuclide with neutron excess.

7. a. **False.** In some radionuclides, following beta decay, the gamma ray is not emitted immediately. The radionuclides before and after emission of the gamma rays are said to be isomers, which have different energy states and half-lives, but the same atomic and mass numbers.

b. **True.**

c. **False.**

d. **True.**

e. **False.** The isomer *before* the release of the gamma ray is said to be metastable.

8. a. **False.** β^+ decay occurs in radionuclides with a neutron deficit.

b. **False.** Radionuclides lose energy and become stable in β^+ decay by a proton changing to a neutron plus a positive electron (known as a positron). The positron is ejected from the nucleus with high energy.

c. **True.**

d. **False.** The conversion of a proton to a neutron results in the atomic mass being conserved.

e. **True.**

9. a. **False.** A radionuclide with a neutron deficit may increase its number of neutrons by capturing an electron from the K-shell, which combines with a proton to form a neutron.

b. **False.** The neutron (no charge) is formed from the combination of a negative electron and a positive proton, leaving no net change in the charge.

c. **True.** The conversion of a proton to a neutron results in the atomic mass being conserved.

d. **True.** Atomic number is equal to the number of protons.

e. **False.** The daughter nuclide emits characteristic X-ray radiation as a result of an electron from an outer shell filling the vacancy in the K-shell.

10. a. **False.** Electromagnetic radiation is identified according to its source. Electrons interacting with a tungsten target, in an X-ray tube, form X-rays. Gamma rays are formed as a result of radioactive decay in the nucleus.

b. **False.** Gamma rays have similar properties to X-rays, both of which have no mass.

c. **True.**

d. **True.** Similar to X-rays, frequency is proportional to photon energy, which is inversely proportional to wavelength.

e. **True.** Gamma rays can interact with an inner-shell electron displacing it from the atom (conversion electron). The vacancy is filled with an electron from the outer shell leading to X-ray emission. This process is known as 'internal conversion.'

11. a. **False.** Beta radiation is made up of electrons. Negative electrons are known as negative beta particles and positive electrons are known as positrons.

b. **True.**

c. **True.**

d. **True.**

e. **False.** Like other secondary electrons, beta rays follow a random path in matter.

12. a. **True.** Like electrons, positrons have a relative atomic mass of 1/1840.

b. **True.** Beta particles are secondary electrons that travel through matter resulting in a trail of ions.

c. **False.** The collision of a positron with a negative electron results in the two charges neutralizing each other and the two masses being converted to energy (annihilation).

d. **True.** The process of annihilation results in the release of gamma photons, which travel in opposite directions to each other.

e. **True.** As these secondary electrons travel through tissue, some of their kinetic energy is transformed to heat energy.

13. a. **True.**

b. **False.** For example, Re-188 is generator produced.

c. **False.** This is a measurement of radiation dose, not activity.

d. **False.** Count rate is proportional to the number of atoms in a sample.

e. **False.** Radioactive decay is a stochastic process; however, within a half-life there is a 50% chance of a particular atom of a radioactive material decaying.

14. a. **True.** This is referred to as the exponential law.

b. **True.** The higher the rate of decay, the higher the number of gamma and beta particles produced.

c. **False.** Some isotopes have multiple decay patterns producing a range of gamma rays. Examples include Ga-67 and I-131.

    d. **False.** The activity of a radionuclide decreases exponentially and hence never reaches zero.

    e. **True.** The number of radioactive atoms in a sample is proportional to the rate of decay.

15. a. **True.**

    b. **False.** The activity of a radioactive sample decreases by equal fractions in equal time intervals (exponential law).

    c. **False.** The degree of radioactivity depends on the quantity of radioactive material at any given moment.

    d. **False.** Although cyclotron-produced radioisotopes generally have short half-lives, some such as Ga-67 and In-111 have longer half-lives than Tc-99m.

    e. **True.**

16. a. **False.** Biological half-life is dependent on the rate of elimination of the radiopharmaceutical from the body.

    b. **True.** A radiopharmaceutical is eliminated from the body by organ-dependent processes such as metabolism (liver) and excretion (kidneys).

    c. **True.** 1/effective half-life = 1/physical half-life + 1/biological half-life.

    d. **False.** The effective half-life is shorter than the biological or physical half-life.

    e. **False.** The biological half-life is dependent on the pharmaceutical agent used, as well as patient factors (e.g. disease process, renal failure) and therefore differs among individuals.

17. a. **False.** The physical half-life is the time taken for a radiopharmaceutical to decay to half its original value.

    b. **False.** The physical half-life is a fixed characteristic of the radiopharmaceutical and is unaffected by factors such as heat and chemical reactions.

    c. **True.** The exponential decay graph can be used to calculate how much activity should be prepared in order to use at a particular time later on.

    d. **False.** The physical half-life is dependent on the decay of the radionuclide and is not influenced by the pharmaceutical agent used.

    e. **False.**

18. a. **True.** The effective half-life is calculated from both the biological and physical half-lives.

    b. **False.** The effective half-life may not depend on renal excretion e.g. Kr-81m, and, even if it does, renal failure results in an increased biological half-life and therefore an increased effective half-life.

    c. **True.** The dose to an organ increases in proportion to the effective half-life.

    d. **True.** This is mainly due to the fact that the biological half-life varies among individuals according to their disease state and physiological factors.

    e. **False.** This will only be the case in those radiopharmaceuticals that are excreted by the biliary system.

19. a. **False.** This would result in high blood pool activity, which may reduce uptake in the target organ.

    b. **True.** The half-life should ideally be a few hours, roughly equal to the time from injection to scanning.

c. **True.** Decay should be to a stable daughter in order to minimize the dose to the patient.

d. **False.** A radionuclide should have a high specific activity, i.e. high activity per unit volume.

e. **False.** Beta particles act as secondary electrons and deposit an unnecessary dose in patients.

20. a. **True.** Below 100 keV, scatter and attenuation within the patient become problematic, e.g. Tl-201.

b. **False.** The pulse height analyser filters out scatter by accepting gamma rays that fall within a small energy window; therefore monoenergetic gamma rays are preferable.

c. **False.** High-energy gamma rays are difficult to collimate and a proportion will also pass straight through the crystal of the gamma camera without being detected.

d. **False.** Low-energy gamma rays are absorbed by the patient and do not reach the gamma camera.

e. **True.** Gamma rays result in the formation of the image, whereas the beta particles deposit an unnecessary dose in the patient.

21. a. **False.** It should only accumulate in the target tissue.

b. **False.** The biological half-life should be suited to the duration of the test but should not be unduly long in order to reduce the dose to the patient.

c. **True.**

d. **False.** The function of the pharmaceutical agent is to concentrate in the target tissue, whereas the radionuclide will emit gamma rays.

e. **True.**

22. a. **False.** The parent compound of Tc-99m is Mo-99, but it is produced following the emission of a negative beta particle. Tc-99m subsequently emits gamma rays to form its isomer Tc-99.

b. **True.** Tc-99m and Tc-99 are isomers and differ in their half-lives and energy states. They have the same atomic and mass numbers.

c. **True.** Tc-99m emits gamma rays with 140 keV, which are suitable for imaging.

d. **True.** TcO_4^- is trapped in the thyroid gland and the salivary glands, but is also taken up by the gastric mucosa or by ectopic gastric mucosa (Meckel's diverticulum).

e. **False.** Tc-99m results in the emission of pure gamma rays.

23. a. **True.**

b. **True.** Increasing the number of holes results in a higher fraction of gamma rays passing through the collimator.

c. **True.** The higher the sensitivity, i.e. the higher the number of gamma rays passing through the collimator to form the image, the lower the amount of radionuclide needed and hence the lower the patient's dose, but this is usually at the expense of the resolution.

d. **False.** Wider holes allow a higher fraction of gamma rays to pass through.

e. **True.** Longer holes result in a narrower angle of acceptance resulting in more gamma rays being stopped by the collimator.

24. a. **True.**
    b. **True.**
    c. **False.** Pinhole collimators, which are used to image superficial organs, e.g. the thyroid, result in an inverted and magnified image. Convergent collimators result in magnification of the image but do not invert it.
    d. **True.** This is especially useful in mobile cameras, where a small crystal can image a large field of view, e.g. the lungs.
    e. **True.** Other factors that improve spatial resolution include longer and narrower holes.

25. a. **False.** The primary function of the collimator is to delineate the gamma source.
    b. **True.** Each photomultiplier consists of a photocathode that absorbs light and emits photoelectrons. These are accelerated towards an anode and multiply on the way by colliding with dynodes.
    c. **True.** Gamma rays as a result of scatter have a low energy, which is filtered out by the pulse height analyser.
    d. **False.** Low-energy gamma rays result from Compton attenuation in the patient and crystal.
    e. **False.** Spatial resolution is improved by using collimators with narrower and longer holes.

26. a. **False.** The crystal used in gamma cameras is usually made up of NaI but is fragile and can be damaged by both water and heat.
    b. **True.** As a result of photoelectric absorption, the crystal absorbs the majority of gamma rays from Tc-99m.
    c. **False.** The absorption of a single gamma photon produces thousands of light photons, which spread out in all directions.
    d. **False.** Using a thicker crystal improves sensitivity but reduces intrinsic resolution.
    e. **True.** A sheet phantom (filled with Co-57) is used to test the detector, which should give a uniform response to a uniform field. A defective photomultiplier is seen as reduced counts, and a cracked crystal shows a linear defect.

27. a. **False.** Intrinsic resolution refers to the camera in the absence of the collimator.
    b. **True.**
    c. **True.** The larger the patient, the greater the amount of attenuation and scatter, resulting in reduced spatial resolution.
    d. **True.** This is made up of lead stripes on a uniform sheet source.
    e. **True.** This usually consists of a tube containing Tc-99m.

28. a. **True.**
    b. **False.** Below 100 keV, the intrinsic sensitivity is almost 100%, above which it depends on the thickness of the crystal.
    c. **True.** Using a thicker crystal improves sensitivity but reduces spatial resolution.
    d. **False.** Sensitivity is measured using a known amount of activity in a small source.
    e. **True.**

29. a. **True**. SPECT results in separation of overlying structures, which results in better visualization of the target tissues.
    b. **False**.
    c. **True**.
    d. **False**. The gamma camera rotates around the patient and only stops for short periods, resulting in a reduced number of gamma photons being detected and hence a lower count level being registered. Some cameras use continuous acquisition modes, but this will just result in an equal number of counts being obtained, not more.
    e. **True**.

30. a. **False**. Following the collision of a positron with an electron, two gamma photons (511 keV) are produced, which travel in opposite directions. The simultaneous detection of these photons along the line of response will lead to the registration of the event.
    b. **True**. The tracer used most commonly is glucose labelled with Fl-18 (18-FDG), which has a very short half-life. Generators can also be used to produce radionuclides, for example the Ge-68/Ga-68 generator.
    c. **True**.
    d. **False**. PET images provide functional and physiological information and are therefore often fused with computed tomography (CT) or magnetic resonance imaging (MRI) to provide anatomical information.
    e. **False**. Scintillation detectors are most commonly made up of bismuth germanate or lutetium yttrium orthosilicate (LYSO), which have a high detection efficiency and are able to absorb and convert photons with 511 keV into light.

Computed tomography – Questions

N. Sheikh-Bahaei

1. Regarding computed tomography (CT) number (CTn):
   a. It represents the linear attenuation coefficient of each tissue
   b. It is directly proportional to μ_{water}
   c. It depends on kV, but not on filtration
   d. It is between 20 and 30 for brain white matter
   e. Air and water can be used for calibration of CTn

2. Regarding the partial volume effect:
   a. A thin high-contrast object at an oblique angle is less visible
   b. Because of the partial volume effect, a small high-contrast object that is smaller than the display pixel size is not visible
   c. It reduces the visibility of low-contrast detail
   d. It depends on the thickness of the tissue
   e. It depends on the thickness of the transaxial slice

3. In CT:
   a. The total number of detectors is around 500–1000 in each row
   b. The gantry cannot tilt in the cranio-caudal direction
   c. A bone algorithm improves the spatial resolution
   d. The anode–cathode axis is perpendicular to the z-axis to reduce the heel effect
   e. The main filter is usually 3 mm of aluminium

4. In CT geometry:
   a. There are typically two focal spots and the smallest is 0.6 mm
   b. The heating capacity is 0.4 MJ
   c. The filter in first-generation scanners was copper to remove high-energy photons and aluminium for low-energy photons
   d. Post-patient collimation is necessary in a multi-slice scanner to get an accurate thickness
   e. A bow tie filter is used to reduce scatter at the periphery of the image

5. Regarding CT generations:
   a. In first-generation scanners, the gantry rotated 360° as well as the single detector
   b. The second-generation scanner is a rotate–translate scanner
   c. In second-generation scanners, the detectors can cover the whole cross-section in one radiation
   d. In third-generation scanners, the patient-to-detector distance is greater than in other generation scanners
   e. In third-generation scanners, data acquisition is continuous

6. Regarding fourth-generation CT scanners:
   a. The dose is less than in other generations
   b. The number of detectors is increased by a factor of 8
   c. They need simpler reconstruction
   d. The calibration can be readjusted through each scanning cycle
   e. They are the best for cardiac imaging

7. Regarding detectors in CT:
   a. The larger the detectors, the better the spatial resolution
   b. They should have negligible afterglow and a narrow dynamic range
   c. In single-slice scanners, the ionization chamber is elongated in the direction of the X-ray beam to increase the efficiency
   d. In multi-slice scanners, the scintillant is often bismuth germanate
   e. Solid detectors are less sensitive but more stable in comparison with gas chambers

8. Regarding CT:
   a. In scanograms, the scatter is high and spatial resolution is poor
   b. CT fluoroscopy is a low kV technique in which the table does not move
   c. In CT fluoroscopy, both the effective dose and the skin dose are less than in normal CT
   d. A scanogram is another name for a scout view
   e. CT fluoroscopy is used for biopsy needle placement

9. Regarding pitch in CT:
   a. The table movement over the slice width is the row pitch in a multi-slice scanner
   b. If the length of area to be scanned is 600 mm and the slice pitch is 2 with a slice thickness of 15 mm, 20 rotations are needed to cover the whole field of view
   c. The beam pitch is usually between 2 and 3 to reduce the patient's dose
   d. The beam pitch is always equal to or smaller than the slice pitch
   e. In 12 rows of 2 mm detectors, the slice thickness could be 1, 2, 4, 6 or 12

10. Which of these statements are true?
    a. The number of measurements for reconstruction is dependent on the number of detectors
    b. Filter back projection is the most common image reconstruction technique used
    c. In filter back projection, the effect of the neighbouring beam on each pixel is directly proportional to their distance
    d. The partial volume effect is greater in spiral CT
    e. Helical/spiral CT needs more heat capacity

11. Regarding spatial resolution:
    a. CT has a better spatial resolution compared with film-screen radiography
    b. It is 3–5 line pairs mm^{-1} in digital imaging
    c. It depends on the width of the projection path
    d. The source-to-detector distance affects unsharpness but not the spatial resolution
    e. If the matrix is 512 × 512 and the field of view is 60 cm, then the spatial resolution would be 4 line pairs mm^{-1}

12. Regarding image quality:
    a. Bone reconstruction will increase the spatial resolution and reduce the noise
    b. Spatial resolution depends on focal spot size
    c. The number of projections sampled in each rotation will affect the spatial resolution
    d. The higher the pitch, the better the spatial resolution
    e. Both contrast resolution and spatial resolution are better in CT than film-screen radiography

13. Regarding noise:
    a. It reduces the contrast resolution of small objects
    b. It reduces the spatial resolution of high-contrast objects
    c. It is inversely proportional to the speed of image acquisition
    d. With a constant patient dose, a higher kV increases the noise and reduces the contrast
    e. A larger matrix increases the noise

14. Regarding slice thickness in CT:
    a. Increasing the slice width increases the noise
    b. Increasing the slice thickness reduces the spatial resolution
    c. Reducing the slice thickness increases the partial volume effect
    d. The slice thickness cannot be less than the detector width
    e. In single-slice CT, the pitch does not affect the noise

15. Regarding noise and the signal-to-noise ratio (SNR) in CT:
    a. SNR is inversely proportional to slice width
    b. SNR is proportional to the square root of mA and kV
    c. The noise becomes more apparent as the window width is reduced
    d. The window width does not affect SNR
    e. Electronic noise is produced by the reconstruction system

16. Which of the following are correct regarding image quality in CT?
    a. Structural noise is the least significant type of noise in CT
    b. Narrowing the window width reveals low-contrast objects
    c. The cone beam effect is more significant with an increasing number of total detectors
    d. 3D reconstruction displays the maximum voxel values along each ray path
    e. A smaller matrix size means less spatial resolution and less noise

17. Regarding artefacts in CT:
    a. Bands of black and white through a cross-section are secondary to motion artefacts
    b. To overcome streak artefacts, a bow tie filter should be used
    c. In beam hardening, the attenuation coefficient decreases at the periphery of the image
    d. The cupping effect is a result of photon starvation
    e. Horizontal streaks across the image can be the effect of photon starvation

18. Which of the following are correct regarding image acquisition in CT?
    a. Multi-slice scanners are more susceptible to ring artefacts
    b. The cone beam effect causes blurry boundaries between high-contrast details
    c. The distance between the X-ray source and the patient will affect spatial resolution

   d. All the detectors in each row in CT are of the same size

   e. A 180° arc is used in cardiac CT for data collection

19. Regarding CT dosimetry:
    a. The CT dose index (CTDI) is dependent on filtering
    b. An increase in kV does not affect the CTDI but increases the dose at a specific point, z (D_z)
    c. At a constant mA, the dose is inversely proportional to pitch
    d. mA affects the CTDI but not D_z (dose at point z)
    e. If the true profile width is equal to a nominal width, CTDI is independent of the slice width

20. Regarding the CT dose index (CTDI):
    a. Practically, the weighted CTDI (CTDI$_w$) is 1/3 CTDI$_{centre}$ + 2/3 CTDI$_{average\ periphery}$
    b. The average absorbed dose is CTDI$_w$ × pitch
    c. The maximum skin dose for a CT head is equal to CTDI$_w$
    d. CTDI is a measure of the dose from a single rotation of the gantry
    e. A pencil ionization chamber is used to measure CTDI

21. Regarding dose in CT:
    a. In a body CT, the maximum skin dose is higher than the weighted CTDI (CTDI$_w$)
    b. CTDI is higher in a CT head than a CT body
    c. CTDI is the best indicator of dose to an individual patient
    d. The skin dose in CT is higher than in prolonged fluoroscopy
    e. CTDI$_{vol}$ is an approximation of the average skin dose

22. Regarding the dose–length product (DLP):
    a. It is dependent on the number of rotations
    b. DLP is defined as weighted CT dose index (CTDI$_w$) × L (scan length)
    c. Collimation does not affect DLP but influences the effective dose
    d. DLP is usually higher for a head CT compared with an abdomen CT
    e. At constant mA, DLP is directly proportional to pitch

23. Which of the following are correct regarding dose–length product (DLP), patient dose and conversion coefficient?
    a. The absorbed dose can be derived from DLP
    b. The conversion coefficient depends on the body region
    c. The conversion coefficient is E (effective dose) × DLP
    d. A high tissue weighting factor reduces the conversion coefficient
    e. The scanner design affects the conversion coefficient

24. Regarding factors influencing the dose:
    a. At a constant mA, a high kV means a higher skin surface dose and a higher absorbed dose
    b. When mA is doubled, the dose is doubled and the noise would be halved
    c. Automated modulation of mA according to the thickness of the patient to keep the noise near constant will reduce the dose compared with the constant mA technique

    d. If the voxel dimensions are halved to keep the signal-to-noise ratio (SNR) constant, the dose will increase eightfold

    e. If the SNR is doubled, the dose would be quadrupled

25. Regarding the dose in single-slice versus multi-slice scanners:
    a. Dose is independent of the slice width in a single-slice scanner
    b. In a single-slice scanner, if mA remains constant, then the thicker the slice width, the lower the dose
    c. In a helical scanner, the field of view affects the dose directly
    d. Post-patient collimation can reduce the dose in a single-slice scanner
    e. The dose is higher in a helical compared with an axial scanner

26. The dose in a multi-slice scanner is higher than in a single-slice scanner because of:
    a. The length of the detector
    b. Overcollimation
    c. A higher pitch
    d. A shorter scanning time
    e. A thinner slice

27. Regarding the CT dose index (CTDI):
    a. $CTDI_{vol}$ is measured in mGy ·
    b. For measurement of the weighted CTDI ($CTDI_w$) for body scanning, a 16 cm diameter phantom is used
    c. The E_{DLP} (normalized effective dose) is measured in mSv mGy^{-1} cm
    d. The effective dose in CT can be calculated using ionizing chambers
    e. If $CTDI_w$ (body) is 10 mGy per 100 mAs; for imaging 25 cm of chest with 150 mAs and a pitch of 1.25, the DLP would be 300 mGy cm

28. In CT, which of these statements are correct?
    a. The effective dose of an abdomen and pelvis CT is nearly ten times that of an abdominal radiograph
    b. The dose in a chest CT is around 2–3 mSv
    c. The lung window is a narrow window centred on a low-level CT number
    d. Tilting the gantry in a head CT will increase the beam hardening artefacts
    e. The most common method of avoiding photon starvation artefacts is mA modulation

29. Which of these artefacts manifest as streak artefacts?
    a. Photon starvation
    b. Inadequate field of view
    c. Partial volume effect
    d. Cone beam effect
    e. Motion

30. Regarding resolution in CT:
    a. Quarter detector offset means the central line of the detector is offset from the centre of rotation by one-quarter of the width of the detector element

b. Interleaved sampling is the effect of the quarter detector offset
c. Quarter detector offset produces a more blurry image
d. A flying focal spot is used to improve the resolution
e. Isotropic resolution means the resolution in the isocentre is always the same

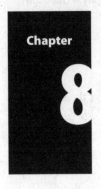
Computed tomography – Answers

1. a. **False.** CT number represents the average linear attenuation coefficient in the voxel.
   b. **False.** $CTn = 1000 \times \mu_t - \mu_w/\mu_w$, where μ_t and μ_w are the attention coefficients of tissue and water, respectively.
   c. **False.** CTn is dependent on:
      - Heterogeneity of the tissue
      - Variation in the attenuation coefficient of each tissue relative to water
      - kV
      - Filtration of the X-ray beam
   d. **True.** CTn of brain white matter = 20–30; CTn of grey matter = 35–45.
   e. **True.** Air and water can be used for calibration.

2. a. **False.** A thin high-contrast object at an oblique angle appears larger.
   b. **False.** A small high-contrast object that is smaller than the displayed pixel size can still be seen.
   c. **True.**
   d. **False.** The partial volume effect depends on the thickness of the transaxial slice, not the tissue.
   e. **True.**

3. a. **True.**
   b. **False.** The gantry can tilt by up to 30° about the vertical.
   c. **True.**
   d. **False.** The anode–cathode axis is parallel to the z-axis to minimize the anode heel effect.
   e. **False.** Filtration typically comprises 6 mm of aluminium. In first-generation scanners, copper was also added to remove low-energy photons.

4. a. **True.**
   b. **False.** The heating capacity is around 4 MJ.
   c. **False.** In first-generation scanners, cooper was used to remove low-energy photons.
   d. **False.** In a single-slice scanner, post-patient collimation is used to reduce scatter when the slice thickness is less than the collimator and also to get an accurate thickness.
   e. **False.** The main purpose of the bow tie filter is to equalize the dose throughout an elliptical shaped body.

5. a. **False.** In first-generation scanners, the X-ray source and single detector both moved across the scanning plane at 180° rotation.
   b. **True.**
   c. **False.** In second-generation scanners, there are around 30 detectors, which are not enough for the whole cross-section.
   d. **False.** In fourth-generation scanners, the patient-to-detector distance is greater than in other generations.
   e. **True.** In third-generation scanners, data collection is continuous for the full 360°.

6. a. **False.** Fourth-generation CT uses rotate–stationary scanners. The advantages are: detector stability, simpler reconstruction and readjustment of calibration through the scanning cycle. The disadvantages are: an increase in the number of detectors by a factor of 6, it is prohibitive in multi-slice CT, and there is a higher dose because of the increased distance between the patient and the detectors.
   b. **False.**
   c. **True.**
   d. **True.**
   e. **False.**

7. a. **False.** For good spatial resolution, the detectors should be small.
   b. **False.** The detectors should have fast response and negligible afterglow and also a wide dynamic range.
   c. **True.**
   d. **True.**
   e. **True.** Solid detectors have a linear response and negligible afterglow. They are very small and stable, but less sensitive in comparison with ionization chambers.

8. a. **False.** In scanograms (topograms), the scatter is minimal and spatial resolution is poor.
   b. **True.** In CT fluoroscopy, the gantry rotates 180° without the table moving, and it is a low kV technique.
   c. **False.** In CT fluoroscopy the effective dose is less but the skin dose is higher because it is confined to a narrow region.
   d. **True.** A scanogram is another name for a scout view.
   e. **True.**

9. a. **True.** Slice pitch = row pitch = table movement/slice width.
   b. **False.** The number of rotations = [600/(2 × 15)] + 2 (extra rotations for start and end points) = 22.
   c. **False.** The beam pitch in CT is between 1 and 2. A pitch above 2 is not acceptable.
   d. **True.** Beam pitch = table movement/collimation length, and slice pitch = table movement/slice width. As the collimation is never smaller than the slice width, the beam pitch is always equal to or smaller than the slice pitch.
   e. **False.** When the detector size is 2 mm, the slice thickness cannot be smaller than 2 mm. The slice thickness could 2, 4, 6 or 12.

10. a. **True.** Number of measurements for reconstruction of the image = number of detectors × number of scans at 360°.
   b. **True.**
   c. **False.** The effect of the neighbouring beam is inversely proportional to the distance.
   d. **False.** The advantages of helical/spiral CT are: high speed, reduced misregistration, continuous data acquisition, a single exposure and reduced partial volume effect. In spiral CT, less contrast medium is required but more heat loading or capacity is needed.
   e. **True.**

11. a. **False.** The spatial resolution in CT is 20 line pairs cm^{-1} while in film-screen radiography it is 8–12 line pairs mm^{-1}
   b. **True.**
   c. **True.** Spatial resolution in CT depends on the following:
   - The matrix and field of view
   - An algorithm: like bone reconstruction, this enhances the edge of high-contrast structures and increases the spatial resolution at the cost of increased noise
   - The width of the projection path, which is affected by focal spot size/source to isocentre and source to detector distance/size of the sensitive area of the detector
   - The number of projections sampled in each rotation. In the z direction, this depends on slice thickness or pitch: the higher the pitch, the less the spatial resolution. This effect is less important in a multi-slice scanner.
   d. **False.**
   e. **True.** Spatial resolution = $1/(2 \times$ pixel size) and pixel size = field of view/matrix = $1/(2 \times 60/512) = 4.3$; therefore, the spatial resolution is around 4 line pairs mm^{-1}.

12. a. **False.** Bone reconstruction enhances the edges of high-contrast structures. It increases the spatial resolution at the cost of increased noise.
   b. **True.** See Q11.
   c. **True.** See Q11.
   d. **False.** See Q11.
   e. **False.** CT has a better contrast resolution compared with film-screen radiography, but the spatial resolution in CT is less.

13. a. **True.** Noise reduces both contrast resolution of small objects and spatial resolution of low-contrast objects.
   b. **False.**
   c. **False.** An increase in speed means fewer incident photons and higher noise, so it is directly proportional to the noise.
   d. **False.** To keep the patient dose constant, when the kV increases the mA will be reduced, but the number of photons detected would still be increased in comparison with a low kV scan and noise will consequently be reduced in relation to signal. However, a high kV reduces the contrast.
   e. **True.** A reduced field of view or increased matrix size = smaller pixels = increased noise.

14. a. **False.** Increasing the slice thickness reduces noise but reduces spatial resolution and increases the partial volume effect at the same time.
    b. **True.**
    c. **False.**
    d. **True.**
    e. **True.** In a single-slice scanner, the pitch does not affect the noise, but it affects spatial resolution and the partial volume effect, while in multi-slice scanners, increasing the pitch increases the noise.

15. a. **False.** The SNR is proportional to the square root of the slice width.
    b. **False.** It is proportional only to the square root of mA.
    c. **True.** Reduction of window width makes noise more apparent but does not change the SNR.
    d. **True.**
    e. **False.** Electronic noise is produced by the measuring system while structural noise is from the reconstruction system.

16. a. **False.** Electronic noise is the least significant type of noise in CT.
    b. **True.**
    c. **True.** The cone beam effect is more significant with an increasing number of slices or number of total detectors.
    d. **False.** In 3D reconstruction, instead of displaying the maximum voxel values along each ray path, the ranges of CT numbers may be displayed with varying degrees of opacity.
    e. **True.**

17. a. **True.**
    b. **False.** To overcome high-attenuation (streak) artefacts, a metal correction algorithm should be used.
    c. **False.** In beam hardening, the low-energy photons are filtered so the attenuation coefficient and CT number decrease in the middle part of the image between high-contrast materials.
    d. **False.** Cupping is the effect of beam hardening.
    e. **True.**

18. a. **False.** In multi-slice scanners, a larger change in sensitivity of the detector is needed to cause ring artefacts, so it is less susceptible.
    b. **True.** Blurry boundaries between high-contrast details results from the cone beam effect.
    c. **True.**
    d. **False.**
    e. **True.**

19. a. **True.** The CTDI depends on mA, kV and filtering, but is independent of the slice width.
    b. **False.**
    c. **True.**
    d. **False.** D_z is proportional to mA, rotation, slice width and 1/pitch.
    e. **True.**

20. a. **True.**
    b. **False.** $CTDI_{vol} = CTDI_w/pitch$ = average absorbed dose within the scan volume.
    c. **True.** Maximum skin dose is equal to $CTDI_w$ for a CT head, but it is 20% higher for a body CT.
    d. **True.**
    e. **True.**

21. a. **True.**
    b. **True.** CTDI: head CT > abdo-pelvis CT > chest CT.
    c. **False.** CTDI measures the dose efficiency. It is mainly for comparison between different models/protocols; it does not measure the dose for individual patients.
    d. **False.** Skin dose: prolonged fluoroscopy > CT > plain film.
    e. **False.**

22. a. **True.** DLP depends on the number of rotations, collimation length and pitch.
    b. **False.** $DLP = CTDI_{vol} \times L$.
    c. **False.**
    d. **True.** DLP: head CT > abdo-pelvis CT > chest CT.
    e. **True.**

23. a. **False.** The effective dose can be derived from DLP.
    b. **True.** The conversion coefficient depends on the body region and scanner design.
    c. **False.** Conversion coefficient = E/DLP.
    d. **False.** A high tissue weighting factor increases the conversion coefficient: it is higher in the abdomen than in the chest and lowest in the head.
    e. **True.**

24. a. **True.**
    b. **False.** mA is in direct relation to the dose but noise is proportional to $\sqrt{mA}$, so the dose will be doubled and the noise will be $\sqrt{2}$.
    c. **True.**
    d. **True.** If the pixels are halved, then the incident photon will be $(1/2)^3$; therefore, for the same signal-to-dose ratio, the dose needs to be eight times higher.
    e. **True.** mA and therefore dose is proportional to $(SNR)^2$; thus, $(SNR \times 2)^2 = 4 \times dose$.

25. a. **True.**
    b. **False.** Slice thickness does not affect the dose if mA remains the same; it means that the noise is higher.
    c. **False.** Neither reconstruction nor the field of view affect the dose directly. They do influence the noise and subsequently the mA.
    d. **False.** Post-patient collimation increases the patient's dose.
    e. **True.**

26. a. **True.**
    b. **True.**
    c. **False.**
    d. **False.**
    e. **True.**

27. a. **False.**
   b. **False.** A 16 cm diameter phantom is used for the head and a 32 cm diameter phantom is used for the body.
   c. **False.** E_{DLP} is measured in mSv mGy^{-1} cm^{-1}. The effective dose is derived from $E_{DLP} \times$ DLP.
   d. **False.** Effective doses in CT can be calculated using special computer programs. A special ionization chamber detector is used to measure CTDI.
   e. **True.** DLP: CTDI$_w$ $\times$ 1/pitch $\times$ length; therefore, CTDI$_w$ for 150 mAs is 15 mGy = 15 $\times$ 1/1.25 $\times$ 25 = 300 mGy cm.

28. a. **True.** The effective dose of an abdomen and pelvis CT is 7 mSv and an abdominal radiograph is 0.6 mSv.
   b. **False.** The effective dose of a chest CT is around 6 mSv.
   c. **False.** Lung window: width 1000, length −500. The wide window, centred on a low CT number, allows a wide range of CT numbers in the lung to be depicted. However, contrast in the soft tissues of the mediastinum and chest wall is poor.
   d. **False.** Strategies to minimize beam hardening artefacts include:
   - patient positioning: for example, tilting the gantry for head scans to avoid imaging through regions of densest bone or dental fillings
   - iterative beam hardening corrections: these may be incorporated into the reconstruction on some scanners. From an initial reconstruction, the image is segmented to identify areas of bone. The beam hardening effects of the bone are modelled and used to pre-correct the data. This process may be repeated iteratively to produce a final image essentially free from beam hardening artefacts. However, the reconstructing time is consequently increased.
   e. **True.** The most common method of avoiding photon starvation artefacts is to employ tube current modulation (or 'mA modulation'). In many modern scanners, the tube current (mA) can be varied as the gantry rotates around the patient. A higher mA is used for the more attenuating projections and a lower mA for the less attenuating projections. The mA to be used is calculated either in advance from analysis of the scout view or during the scan via a feedback system from the detector.

29. a. **True.**
   b. **True.**
   c. **True.**
   d. **True.**
   e. **True.**

30. a. **True.**
   b. **True.**
   c. **False.** Interleaved sampling gives a finer angular spacing of projections. This helps to reduce artefacts that arise when the projections are too sparsely spaced.
   d. **True.** The position of the focal spot on the anode is varied rapidly in the transaxial plane. This can be used to effectively double the number of projections sampled and will improve resolution.
   e. **False.** Isotropic resolution means the resolution is the same in all directions.

Imaging with ultrasound – Questions

T. Matys

1. Regarding the properties of ultrasound:
   a. Ultrasound propagates through tissue as a longitudinal wave
   b. The velocity of the ultrasound wave is equal to the velocity of the particles of the tissue through which it propagates
   c. The wavelength of ultrasound in tissue in the range of frequencies used in diagnostic imaging is 1–5 mm
   d. An ultrasound wave undergoes reflection and refraction but not Rayleigh scattering
   e. Attenuation of the ultrasound wave by 10 dB corresponds to a tenfold decrease in ultrasound intensity

2. Ultrasound velocity:
   a. Is equal to the ultrasound frequency divided by the wavelength
   b. Increases with frequency in a given medium
   c. Is proportional to the square root of the material density
   d. Is higher in compressible materials
   e. Is lower in tissues with a higher fat or water content

3. Which of the following are true about acoustic impedance?
   a. It is measured in $kg\ m^{-2}$
   b. The acoustic impedance of fat is lower than most other tissues
   c. The acoustic impedance of air is almost zero
   d. It is independent of temperature
   e. The intensity of ultrasound is directly proportional to the acoustic impedance and to the wave amplitude

4. Concerning the reflection of ultrasound waves:
   a. Specular reflection occurs when the size of the reflector is much larger than the ultrasound wavelength
   b. The angle of specular reflection depends on the differences in acoustic impedance of tissues forming the boundary and is described by Snell's law
   c. For a normal angle of incidence, approximately 30–40% of ultrasound is transmitted at an interface between bone and soft tissue
   d. The degree of ultrasound reflection at an interface between different soft tissues (for example, fat–muscle interface) is up to 10%
   e. The echotexture of the liver parenchyma is due to scattering

5. Regarding ultrasound refraction:
   a. The angle of refraction depends on the velocities of ultrasound in the media on both sides of the boundary
   b. Ultrasound traversing an interface between muscle and bone will bend towards the normal
   c. The critical angle is the angle of incidence at which the refracted beam travels parallel to the boundary
   d. Refraction plays an important role in the phenomenon of acoustic enhancement behind a fluid-filled structure
   e. Refraction is one of the principal causes of artefacts in ultrasound imaging

6. Concerning the attenuation of ultrasound:
   a. In contrast to the attenuation of X-rays, it is not an exponential process
   b. It is mostly due to loss of energy from the primary beam due to scattering and reflection
   c. In a particular medium, it depends on the frequency of the ultrasound
   d. The attenuation coefficient of water is similar to that of non-clotted blood
   e. A thickness of tissue equal to the half-value layer (HVL) attenuates the ultrasound beam by 3 dB

7. Concerning the construction of a single ultrasound transducer probe:
   a. It contains a piezoelectric crystal usually made of lead zirconate titanate (PZT)
   b. During the manufacturing process, the crystal is heated above the Curie point and is polarized by an external voltage, which is maintained until the temperature falls below the Curie point
   c. At the resonant frequency, the transducer produces ultrasound of a wavelength equal to half the thickness of the crystal
   d. To match the properties of the piezoelectric element and the tissue, a matching layer is applied to the surface of the PZT with the acoustic impedance being a geometric mean of PZT and tissue, and thickness equal to half the wavelength produced at the resonant frequency
   e. The acoustic impedance of the backing layer used to dampen the transducer needs to be identical to that of the piezoelectric crystal

8. Concerning the Q factor of an ultrasound transducer:
   a. A low Q transducer has a narrow bandwidth
   b. A heavily damped transducer has a low Q factor
   c. A low Q transducer can achieve better axial resolution than a high Q transducer of the same frequency
   d. High Q transducers are preferred for continuous-wave imaging
   e. Continuous-wave Doppler imaging requires a receiving transducer that is lightly damped

9. Regarding an ultrasound beam produced by a single transducer:
   a. It initially propagates as a plane wave with a diameter similar to the transducer diameter
   b. The length of the near field is proportional to the radius of the transducer and the ultrasound wavelength

   c. The area where the beam starts to diverge is termed the Fresnel region

   d. The angle of divergence is proportional to the ultrasound wavelength

   e. A beam from a single transducer cannot be focused, as focusing is only possible in array transducers

10. Concerning resolution in ultrasound imaging:

   a. Azimuthal resolution is the ability to separate two objects lying along the line of the ultrasound beam

   b. Axial resolution is equal to twice the spatial pulse length (SPL)

   c. Axial resolution can be improved by using a transducer with a high frequency and a low Q

   d. Azimuthal resolution is independent of depth

   e. In the focal area, axial and azimuthal resolutions are equal

11. Regarding the operation of array transducers:

   a. To obtain a focused beam, the innermost element of the annular array is energized first

   b. Focusing in a linear array is achieved by first energizing the outermost elements of the active group

   c. The shorter the time delay between energizing the elements of the array, the shorter the focal distance

   d. In contrast to annular probes, array transducers do not give rise to grating lobes

   e. An ultrasound beam formed from a linear array may be steered from side to side by using the apodization technique

12. Concerning ultrasound scanning modes:

   a. The returning ultrasound echoes are depicted in the A-mode as a series of dots whose brightness is proportional to the echo amplitude

   b. Real-time B-mode imaging requires a mechanical sector scanner or an array transducer

   c. In the M-mode, the echoes are displayed as lines of bright dots on a time line

   d. 'Duplex scanning' refers to simultaneous B-mode and M-mode imaging

   e. 3D scanning always requires a dedicated 3D probe that is able to steer the ultrasound beam in two orthogonal directions

13. Regarding real-time B-mode imaging:

   a. A typical number of scan lines in B-mode imaging of the abdomen is 256

   b. To avoid flicker, the frame rate should be at least 20–25 frames per second (fps)

   c. The maximum scan line density at a frame rate of 25 fps and a pulse repetition frequency (PRF) of 2 kHz is 50

   d. The maximum depth of view at a frame rate of 30 fps and a scan line density of 100 is approximately 33 cm

   e. The maximum achievable frame rate with a line density of 100 and a depth of view of 15 cm is approximately 50 fps

14. Concerning tissue harmonic imaging (THI):

   a. It usually uses echoes with frequencies that are integral multiples of the fundamental frequency

   b. It requires a narrow bandwidth transducer

   c. The basal frequency can be suppressed by using a pulse inversion technique

   d. The azimuthal resolution suffers in comparison with standard ultrasound imaging techniques

   e. Reverberation artefacts and side lobe artefacts are reduced

15. Regarding the Doppler effect:
   a. It is a change in the velocity of the sound reflected from a moving object
   b. For an object moving away from the transducer, the Doppler shift is negative
   c. For a given angle of insonation, the Doppler shift frequency depends only on the original sound frequency and the velocity of the reflector
   d. The Doppler shift frequencies in medical ultrasound imaging are in the audible range
   e. With other parameters being equal, the maximum Doppler shift will be recorded when a transducer is perpendicular to the object path

16. In relation to continuous-wave Doppler imaging:
   a. It uses a transducer with two slightly angled crystals
   b. A good range resolution can be achieved
   c. High velocities can be measured accurately
   d. It cannot be used in pregnancy due to the high energy deposited by the continuous ultrasound wave
   e. A continuous Doppler signal is usually presented to the user as an audible sound

17. Concerning pulsed-wave Doppler imaging:
   a. It uses a single transducer that alternates between transmission and reception
   b. It shows a 2D map of flow with the flow towards the transducer demonstrated in red, and away from the transducer in blue
   c. It allows the measurement of high-velocity flow
   d. Range resolution is achieved through a range gating
   e. The maximum depth of sampling depends on the pulse repetition frequency (PRF)

18. Regarding aliasing in pulsed-wave Doppler imaging:
   a. It occurs when the Doppler shift frequency exceeds 2 PRF (pulse repetition frequency)
   b. It limits the range of velocities than can accurately be measured to $1.5–2\,\mathrm{m\ s^{-1}}$
   c. The risk of aliasing is higher at higher Doppler frequencies
   d. It can be reduced by using a higher PRF, lowering the frequency or increasing the angle of insonation
   e. The problem of aliasing can partially be overcome by using a high PRF mode

19. Concerning parameters and indices used in Doppler imaging:
   a. To detect slow flow, it may be necessary to increase the Doppler frequency or decrease the pulse repetition frequency (PRF)
   b. Increasing the wall filter is helpful in the detection of slow flow
   c. The signal-to-noise ratio (SNR) may be improved by using a high-pass filter
   d. The resistance index (RI) is calculated as (peak systolic flow – end diastolic flow)/(peak systolic flow)
   e. Examples of vessels with a low RI include the renal artery, the uterine artery in pregnancy and the external carotid artery

20. Regarding colour flow imaging (CFI) and power Doppler imaging:
    a. Image acquisition in CFI is based on the continuous-wave Doppler
    b. CFI is not susceptible to aliasing
    c. On modern ultrasound equipment, the frame rate achieved in colour flow mode is the same as the frame rate in the corresponding pure B-mode imaging
    d. In power Doppler imaging, the sensitivity to motion is not dependent on the Doppler angle
    e. CFI is more susceptible to flash artefacts than power Doppler imaging

21. Concerning artefacts in ultrasound imaging:
    a. A slice thickness artefact may result in the appearance of low-level echoes in small cysts
    b. Comet-tail artefacts differ from ring-down artefacts by the banded appearance of the latter
    c. Compound imaging helps visualize renal calculi
    d. The artefact when liver appears to lie on the upper side of the diaphragm is an example of a reverberation artefact
    e. A clutter artefact is found at the interface between Fresnel and Fraunhofer zones, where the ultrasound beam starts to diverge

22. Microbubbles used as ultrasound contrast agents:
    a. Have a gaseous core
    b. Are similar in diameter to neutrophils
    c. Have resonance frequency in a low MHz range
    d. Mainly accumulate in the blood pool
    e. Can be destroyed by ultrasound waves

23. Concerning detection of microbubbles and their applications:
    a. The main use for microbubbles is to enhance Doppler ultrasound imaging
    b. As microbubbles are quickly destroyed by insonation, they can only be imaged intermittently
    c. Stimulated acoustic emission (SAE) utilizes high-energy Doppler pulses
    d. Characterization of liver lesions with microbubbles is usually based on their enhancement pattern
    e. Microbubbles can be used for targeted drug delivery

24. Concerning perfluorocarbon nanoparticles as ultrasound contrast agents:
    a. Similarly to microbubbles, they have a gaseous core but are smaller in size ($<1\,\mu m$)
    b. They have a longer half-life in comparison with microbubbles
    c. Like microbubbles, they exhibit non-linear resonance with the production of harmonics
    d. They show a strong acoustic signal while in the blood pool
    e. They have the potential to be used as multi-modality contrast agents

25. Regarding electrical safety and quality assurance (QA) in ultrasound:
    a. Electrical safety tests of the ultrasound unit should be performed annually
    b. QA of the ultrasound unit should be performed semi-annually

   c. The resolution in B-mode imaging may be tested with a string phantom
   d. Phantoms used for B-mode imaging are usually filled with distilled water
   e. The power output of the transducer may be measured with a radiation force
      balance

26. Concerning safety limits and indices used in ultrasound:
   a. The time-averaged ultrasound intensity should nowhere exceed $100 \, \text{mW cm}^{-2}$
   b. The total sound energy (intensity × dwell time) should nowhere
      exceed $100 \, \text{J cm}^{-2}$
   c. The thermal index (TI) is the ratio of the power emitted to the power required to
      increase the whole body temperature by $1°C$
   d. The mechanical index (MI) is the peak rarefaction pressure divided by the square
      root of the ultrasound frequency
   e. Both TI and MI must always be displayed on the ultrasound control panel

27. Concerning the thermal effects of ultrasound:
   a. Potential sources of heating are the absorption of ultrasound waves and heat
      produced at the transducer surface
   b. A temperature rise of less than $1°C$ is considered to present no hazard to human
      tissue including the embryo and fetus, even if maintained indefinitely
   c. According to International Standards IEC (2007), the maximum temperature of the
      probe in contact with the patient should not exceed $43°C$ when used internally, or
      $50°C$ when used externally
   d. Doppler techniques pose greater heating risks when compared with B-mode
      imaging
   e. Spectral Doppler poses less heating risk compared with colour flow imaging

28. Concerning the non-thermal effects of ultrasound:
   a. In general, non-inertial cavitation is not a big problem in ultrasound
   b. The risk of cavitation is increased in the presence of microbubble contrast media
   c. In the presence of microbubbles, there is a risk of cavitation while scanning with a
      mechanical index (MI) in excess of 1.0
   d. Organs at risk of cavitation-related damage in the absence of contrast media include
      the intestine and lungs both in the prenatal and postnatal period
   e. Acoustic streaming has the potential to cause tissue damage with an MI
      above 2.0

29. Regarding the recommendations of the British Medical Ultrasound Society for obstetric
   and neonatal ultrasound:
   a. In obstetric scanning up to 10 weeks after the last menstrual period, the operator
      should monitor the thermal index for bone (TIB)
   b. There are no time restrictions on scanning with a thermal index (TI) <1.0
   c. Scanning of the embryo or fetus is not recommended, however briefly,
      with a TI >3.0
   d. General neonatal scanning is not recommended, however briefly, with a TI >3.0
   e. In neonates, the possibility of lung or intestine damage occurs with a mechanical
      index (MI) >0.7

30. Regarding the recommendations of the British Medical Ultrasound Society for non-obstetric, non-neonatal ultrasound:
    a. Scanning of the eye is not recommended with a thermal index (TI) >1.0, however briefly
    b. There are no time restrictions on scanning with a TI <1.0
    c. Scanning of the central nervous system is not recommended with a TI >3.0, and a general ultrasound examination with a TI >6.0
    d. Consent is required from patients scanned by ultrasound trainees only in the case of transvaginal ultrasound
    e. It is recommended that the total time of the examination performed by ultrasound trainees is normally no more than triple that needed to carry out a diagnostic scan

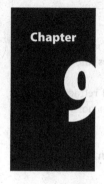
1. a. **True.** This means that local movement of the tissue particles is in the same direction as the wave propagation.
   b. **False.** The velocity of the ultrasound wave is independent of the velocity of the particles of the medium.
   c. **False.** It ranges from approximately 0.77 mm (at 2 MHz frequency) to 0.1 mm (at 15 MHz frequency).
   d. **False.** It undergoes all these processes. Rayleigh scattering occurs when a wave is scattered from small structures with dimensions less than the ultrasound wavelength, such as red blood cells or microbubbles.
   e. **True.** 10 dB (1 Bel) corresponds to a change by one order of magnitude.

2. a. **False.** It is a product of the frequency and wavelength.
   b. **False.** Velocity in a given medium is virtually independent of the frequency. With velocity being constant, an increase in the frequency causes a proportional decrease in wavelength.
   c. **False.** It is inversely proportional to the square root of the material density.
   d. **False.** Ultrasound travels faster in stiff, non-compressible media.
   e. **True.** The velocity of ultrasound in fat and water is lower than in an average soft tissue.

3. a. **False.** The acoustic impedance is a product of ultrasound velocity (in m s^{-1}) and density of the medium (in kg m^{-3}). Therefore, its unit is kg m^{-2} s^{-1}, which is also termed *rayl* after Lord Rayleigh.
   b. **True.** The lower velocity of ultrasound in fat combined with fat being of lower density leads to a lower acoustic impedance.
   c. **True.** This is mainly due to its low density.
   d. **False.** It changes with temperature as the material density and stiffness may change.
   e. **False.** It is proportional to the acoustic impedance and to the square of the amplitude.

4. a. **True.**
   b. **False.** The angle of specular reflection is, by definition, equal to the angle of incidence. Snell's law governs the process of refraction.
   c. **False.** Approximately 30–40% is reflected, and 60–70% is transmitted.
   d. **False.** Only up to 1–2% is reflected.
   e. **True.** Hence, the echotexture of the liver is independent of the sonication angle.

5. a. **True.** The ratio of sines of the angles of incidence and refraction is equal to the ratio of velocities in the two tissues forming the boundary. This is known as Snell's law. `

   b. **False.** The velocity of ultrasound in bone is higher, so the angle of refraction will be larger than the angle of incidence. The beam will bend away from normal (line perpendicular to the boundary).

   c. **True.** The angle of refraction in this case equals 90°.

   d. **False.** Acoustic enhancement is an attenuation artefact. Refraction does not play a role here.

   e. **True.** It may change the apparent position of objects (misregistration) and cause critical angle shadowing at interfaces that are at steep angles to the direction of the ultrasound beam (such as the lateral margins of well-defined structures).

6. a. **False.** The attenuation of ultrasound is also exponential.

   b. **False.** Attenuation is mostly caused by energy absorption by frictional and viscous forces in the medium, with some contribution from scattering and partial reflection.

   c. **True.** The attenuation coefficient of most tissues increases linearly with the frequency, and for soft tissues is typically in the range of 0.3–0.6 dB cm^{-1} MHz^{-1}.

   d. **False.** Water attenuates ultrasound waves to a lesser degree than blood.

   e. **True.** In the logarithmic scale, log $0.5 = 0.3$ Bel $= 3$ dB.

7. a. **True.**

   b. **True.** This orientates the internal dipoles in one direction, giving the crystal its piezoelectric properties. Once the crystal is cooled below the Curie temperature, this orientation is preserved, even in the absence of an external voltage. Heating above the Curie point in the absence of an external voltage would result in destruction of this polarization and elimination of the piezoelectric properties.

   c. **False.** The wavelength produced at the resonant frequency is double the crystal thickness.

   d. **False.** The thickness of the matching plate equals a quarter of the wavelength.

   e. **False.** In this case, all the sound energy would be completely absorbed in the backing layer. Therefore, a backing layer of impedance slightly lower than that of the PZT is used.

8. a. **False.** As the Q factor is the ratio of the resonant frequency to the transducer bandwidth, a low Q value indicates a wide bandwidth.

   b. **True.** A heavily damped transducer produces a pulse of short duration. The shorter the pulse, the wider the spectrum of frequencies produced (bandwidth). Therefore, a heavily damped transducer has a low Q factor.

   c. **True.** A low Q transducer is highly damped and produces a pulse of short duration and therefore of low spatial pulse length (SPL). The shorter the SPL, the better the axial resolution.

   d. **True.** Continuous-wave imaging requires a transducer with high persistence of sound ('ringing'). Such a transducer needs to be lightly damped, and therefore of a high Q factor.

   e. **True.** A high Q transducer has a narrow bandwidth, which is optimal for detection of the relatively small frequency changes caused by the blood flow.

9. a. **True**. This is because every point on the transducer surface produces a spherical wavelet (as described by Huygens' principle); these wavelets undergo constructive and destructive interference producing a planar wave front. This part of the beam is called a 'near field'.
   b. **False**. It is proportional to the squared radius of the transducer and inversely proportional to wavelength; the near field extends further in the case of big transducers emitting high-frequency ultrasound.
   c. **False**. The beam starts to diverge in the far field (Fraunhofer region). The Fresnel region is another name for the near field.
   d. **True**. The sine of this angle is proportional to the ratio of wavelength and transducer diameter. Therefore, a large transducer of high frequency has a less divergent beam in the far field.
   e. **False**. It cannot be focused electronically; however, it can be focused to one set depth using a curved piezoelectric crystal or a plastic acoustic lens at the transducer face.

10. a. **False**. This is a definition of axial (depth) resolution. Azimuthal (lateral) resolution is the ability to resolve two objects lying side by side at the same depth.
    b. **False**. Axial resolution equals half of the SPL, where SPL is the product of wavelength and number of cycles in the ultrasound pulse.
    c. **True**. Higher frequency equals shorter wavelength, while a damped transducer produces a shorter pulse. Both decrease the SPL and therefore improve axial resolution.
    d. **False**. Azimuthal resolution is dependent on the beam width, which varies with depth. For an unfocused transducer, the beam is narrowest, and resolution best, within the near field–far field interface. For a focused transducer, the best resolution is achieved at the focal region.
    e. **False**. Axial resolution is a component of pulse length, while azimuthal resolution is a component of beam width. As the beam width is larger than the pulse length, the azimuthal resolution is always worse.

11. a. **False**. The outermost element is energized first and the innermost element last.
    b. **True**.
    c. **False**. A short focal distance is obtained by using a long delay between energizing the outer- and innermost elements of the active group.
    d. **False**. Grating lobes are weak replicas of the main ultrasound beam, which are unique to array transducers. They are caused by the regular, periodic spacing of the array elements, and arise when the size of the individual elements is larger than half the wavelength. Subdicing (dividing array elements into parts smaller than 0.5λ) may be used to prevent their formation.
    e. **False**. Apodization is a technique used to prevent side lobe formation by applying less power to the outermost elements. Beam steering is achieved by energizing elements in succession beginning from one edge of the active group.

12. a. **False**. They are depicted as vertical lines with an amplitude proportional to the echo strength on a time scale. A series of dots varying in brightness along multiple scan lines is used in B-mode imaging.
    b. **True**.

   c. **True.**

   d. **False.** It refers to simultaneous B-mode and spectral (pulsed-wave) Doppler imaging.

   e. **False.** It can also be performed with a 2D probe using a freehand technique. However, the position of the probe needs to be constantly registered, for example using optical or magnetic tracking.

13. a. **False.** Such a high number of lines is unnecessary, as the lateral resolution is limited anyway. A typical line density is about 100 or slightly more as a compromise between achievable frame rate and scanning depth.

   b. **True.** The limit of temporal resolution of a human eye is about 40 ms, so ideally the frame rate should be above 25 fps. Below 20 fps, flicker (seeing images as separate in time) becomes obvious.

   c. **False.** With a PRF of 2 kHz, an ultrasound pulse is sent 2000 times per second. If 25 frames are to be obtained per second, each of them can have $2000/25 = 80$ lines.

   d. **False.** In 1 s, ultrasound needs to travel double the distance d (from the probe to the depth of view and then back) as many times as the number of scan lines multiplied by frame rate. Therefore, it travels a total distance of $2 \times d \times$ frame rate $\times$ number of scan lines with an average velocity of 1540 m s^{-1}. Therefore, the depth of field can be calculated as $d = 1540/(2 \times$ frame rate $\times$ number of scan lines$) = 1540/(2 \times 30 \times 100) = 1540/6000 \approx 0.25$ (m).

   e. **True.** As per the above equation, the frame rate can be calculated as $1540/(2 \times$ depth of view $\times$ number of scan lines$) = 1540/30 \approx 50$ (fps).

14. a. **True.** Usually, the second harmonic ($2f_0$) reaches a useful amplitude and is used, but super-harmonics ($3f_0$, $4f_0$) can also be recorded with modern transducers.

   b. **False.** Harmonic imaging requires a wide bandwidth transducer, which has the functionality to transmit at f_0 and receive at $2f_0$ (or higher multiples).

   c. **True.** If every other pulse is inverted, odd harmonics (including the basal frequency) can be suppressed.

   d. **False.** The azimuthal (lateral) resolution is improved due to a narrower beam width.

   e. **True.** This is one of the main advantages of using THI.

15. a. **False.** It is a change in the frequency of the sound reflected from a moving object (known as the Doppler shift frequency).

   b. **True.** The recorded frequency will be lower than the original frequency.

   c. **False.** It also depends on the velocity of sound in a given medium according to the following equation:

$$\Delta f = 2f_0 \frac{v}{c} \cos\theta$$

where f_0 is the original frequency, v is the velocity of the object, c is the velocity of sound and θ is the angle of insonation.

   d. **True.** They are in the frequency range of 100 Hz–8 kHz.

   e. **False.** As the recorded Doppler shift is proportional to the cosine of the angle of insonation (the angle between the object path and the transducer), no Doppler shift would be recorded in this case ($\theta = 90°$; $\cos 90° = 0$). The maximum change in frequency would be seen by a transducer parallel to the object path ($\theta = 0°$; $\cos 0° = 1$).

16. a. **True.** It uses two separate crystals with overlapping beams, which act as a receiver and a transmitter.
    b. **False.** There is no depth discrimination.
    c. **True.** This is the main advantage of the continuous-wave Doppler.
    d. **False.** Monitoring the fetal heartbeat is one of its main applications.
    e. **True.** A continuous-wave Doppler is mainly used in simple handheld systems that present the signal this way. The original frequency is removed from the received frequency leaving the Doppler shift ('beat') in the audible range. The pitch of the sound is proportional to the velocity of the object.

17. a. **True.**
    b. **False.** A pulsed-wave Doppler displays spectral information about flow in a specific sample volume against time (sonogram). Colour flow imaging displays a 2D map of the flow.
    c. **False.** The main shortcoming of the pulsed-wave Doppler is a limited range of measured velocities due to aliasing, as governed by the Nyquist limit.
    d. **True.** The transducer sends a Doppler pulse and waits for the returning echoes. The apparatus only accepts the echoes arising in the specified sampling volume that arrive within a specific time-of-flight window.
    e. **True.** As in the standard B-mode imaging, there needs to be sufficient time for the ultrasound pulse to reach the sampling depth and return to the transducer. Therefore, maximum sampling depth is $0.5 \times c/\text{PRF}$ (where c is the speed of sound).

18. a. **False.** According to the Nyquist criterion, the waveform measured (shift frequency in this case) needs to be sampled at least twice in each period (time between pulses). Therefore, aliasing occurs when the Doppler shift exceeds half of the sampling frequency (PRF), not double.
    b. **True.**
    c. **True.** At higher frequencies, the Doppler shift (which is proportional to frequency) will be larger and more likely to exceed 0.5 PRF.
    d. **True.** At higher PRF, the Doppler shift that can be measured without aliasing is proportionally higher. Lowering the frequency or increasing the angle of insonation decreases the Doppler shift frequency, so it is less likely to exceed the Nyquist criterion.
    e. **True.** In this mode, the next Doppler pulse is sent before the echo from the previous pulse is received. This allows measuring of higher flow velocities, but introduces range ambiguity (loss of range resolution).

19. a. **True.** An increase in Doppler frequency results in a larger frequency shift, which is easier to detect. Decreasing the PRF increases the sensitivity to small frequency shifts.
    b. **False.** The wall filter (high-pass filter) eliminates frequencies below a certain value and is used to eliminate low-frequency signals caused by movement of the vessel wall. However, low-frequency shifts from slow flow are also eliminated. Therefore, to improve sensitivity to slow flow, the wall filter needs to be reduced.
    c. **False.** It can be improved by a low-pass filter that allows only frequencies below a certain threshold to pass, and cuts off high frequencies. As noise is usually high frequency, this improves SNR.

   d. **True.** Another important parameter is the pulsatility index (PI) defined as (peak systolic flow – minimum flow)/(time-averaged maximum flow).

   e. **False.** The internal, not external, carotid artery is of low resistance.

20. a. **False.** CFI uses pulsed-wave Doppler acquisition. Multiple pulses are sent over multiple lines and Doppler shifts are obtained from multiple gates along these lines. Information is presented on a 2D map of flow usually superimposed on a B-mode picture, with colour-coded direction of flow. To speed up data acquisition and processing, phase-shift autocorrelation or time domain correlation is used together with faster analysis algorithms.

   b. **False.** The same Nyquist criterion applies as with spectral pulsed-wave Doppler imaging.

   c. **False.** The frame rate in CFI is always lower than in pure B-mode imaging, as multiple pulses (typically 2–20) are sent for each scan line. The Doppler pulses will also need to be interleaved with B-mode imaging pulses, further decreasing the frame rate.

   d. **True.** Power Doppler (energy Doppler) imaging ignores information about the direction and velocity of flow and displays information dependent only on the flow amplitude. This does not change significantly with the angle of insonation.

   e. **False.** As the name implies, flash artefacts are bursts of signal resulting from the motion of tissue. As power Doppler imaging is more sensitive to motion, flash artefacts are more likely to occur.

21. a. **True.** This is due to the ultrasound beam having a specified thickness in the elevation plane (perpendicular to the scan plane). If this thickness is comparable with the size of the cyst, the image may contain echoes from overlapping adjacent tissue. This is similar to partial volume artefacts in computed tomography (CT) imaging, and can be reduced by using a transducer that is able to focus in the elevation plane.

   b. **False.** The former have a characteristic banded appearance.

   c. **False.** Compound imaging is a technique in which an electronically steered beam acquires several overlapping scans from different angles. This helps eliminate artefacts and improves visualization of structures with curved and irregular borders. However, it also eliminates acoustic shadowing, which in this case is a helpful diagnostic clue.

   d. **False.** It is an example of a mirror image artefact (double reflection).

   e. **False.** Clutter is an unwanted signal appearing in the near field close to the transducer surface, caused by vibration of the piezoelectric element and side lobes. It is greatly reduced in harmonic imaging.

22. a. **True.** The core is either air or inert gas (e.g. nitrogen, perfluoropropane, perfluorocarbon) encapsulated in an albumin or lipid shell.

   b. **False.** The diameter of microbubbles is usually 1–4 μm (up to 7 μm), so they are slightly smaller or comparable in size to red blood cells (6–8 μm) and much smaller than neutrophils (12–15 μm). This allows them to cross pulmonary capillaries and produce systemic enhancement after intravenous injection.

c. **True.** Their resonance frequency happens to fall within the range of frequencies used in clinical ultrasound, which is why they are useful in imaging.

d. **True.** However, certain microbubbles can also be taken up by the reticular endothelial system (RES) of the liver and spleen (passive targeting).

e. **True.** Ultrasound waves of high energy cause disruption and collapse of the microbubbles.

23. a. **False.** Due to their high degree of echogenicity, microbubbles indeed enhance the Doppler signal ('Doppler rescue'), which was the original application of these agents, and sometimes continues to be used in transcranial imaging. However, the main application is currently in contrast-specific imaging techniques utilizing non-linear resonance and production of harmonic frequencies.

b. **False.** Real-time imaging with a low mechanical index (MI) is possible.

c. **True.** SAE is the appearance of a random colour pattern when microbubbles burst after insonation with high-energy Doppler pulses. According to the guidelines of the European Federation of Societies for Ultrasound in Medicine and Biology, high MI techniques are not routinely recommended due to a difficult examination technique and the superiority of real-time, low MI imaging.

d. **True.** Scanning with a low MI allows characterization of the lesion enhancement and washout in the arterial and portal phases in real time, and has almost completely superseded high MI techniques (SAE).

e. **True.** They can be laden with drugs and caused to burst by insonation at a specific target site.

24. a. **False.** Nanoparticles have a non-gaseous core (perfluorocarbon emulsion) enclosed in a lipid shell.

b. **True.** They stay in circulation longer as their liquid composition renders them more resistant to mechanical stress.

c. **False.** They do not demonstrate a non-linear response and do not produce harmonics.

d. **False.** They have a low intrinsic echogenicity and cause detectable ultrasound enhancement only after accumulation. Therefore, they can be specifically targeted (e.g. to fibrin in thrombi) and imaged at the target site without any interference from the blood pool.

e. **True.** They can be additionally labelled with technetium for detection by single-photon emission CT (SPECT), or with gadolinium for magnetic resonance imaging (MRI) detection. Thanks to their fluorine content, ^{19}F spectroscopy is also possible.

25. a. **True.**

b. **False.** The Royal College of Radiologists recommends in its 'Standards for Ultrasound Equipment' that testing should be performed annually or biannually.

c. **False.** Resolution is usually tested using a test object containing a set of filament targets in a tissue-mimicking material phantom. A string phantom is used for testing the velocity in a Doppler mode.

d. **False.** They need to be filled with a material in which the speed of sound ($1540\ \text{m s}^{-1}$), attenuation ($0.5\ \text{dB cm}^{-1}\ \text{MHz}^{-1}$) and density ($1050\ \text{kg m}^{-3}$) are close to that in a soft tissue.

e. **True.** The ultrasound emitted from a transducer exerts a force proportional to the output power, which can be 'weighed' on a special balance. A power of 1 W corresponds to approximately 68 mg.

26. a. **True.** This is approximately 1000 times greater than the typical intensity in the focal region.
   b. **False.** It should not exceed $50\,\mathrm{J\,cm^{-2}}$.
   c. **False.** TI applies to the temperature rise in the insonated tissue, not the whole body.
   d. **True.**
   e. **False.** They need to be displayed if the equipment is capable of exceeding a TI or MI of 1.0 in the selected scanning mode (B-mode, spectral Doppler, etc.). In such cases, the indices must be displayed regardless of their value (i.e. even if they are below 1.0).

27. a. **True.**
   b. **False.** According to the British Medical Ultrasound Society, a diagnostic exposure that produces a maximum temperature rise of no more than 1.5°C above normal physiological levels (37°C) may be used clinically without reservation on thermal grounds.
   c. **False.** The temperature of a probe touching the patient either externally or internally should be limited to 43°C. The 50°C temperature limit applies to a probe running in air.
   d. **True.** Doppler imaging involves greater ultrasound intensities.
   e. **False.** There is a higher risk of heating in spectral Doppler as the beam is held in a fixed position.

28. a. **True.** Non-inertial (stable) cavitation is an oscillation of a pre-existing bubble subject to a pressure wave. It develops over several cycles and would require insonation with a continuous ultrasound wave held in one position, which rarely happens in practice. Inertial (transient) cavitation (growth and collapse of a bubble within a few cycles creating shock waves and an extreme local temperature rise) has more potential for damage.
   b. **True.**
   c. **False.** Such a risk exists at an MI above 0.7.
   d. **False.** In an aerated lung, there is indeed a risk of cavitation-induced haemorrhage (e.g. during transoesophageal scanning). As the fetal lung is not aerated, it is not prone to such damage.
   e. **False.** Acoustic streaming (movement of fluid along an ultrasound beam, or 'quartz wind') is unlikely to cause adverse effects.

29. a. **False.** The thermal index for soft tissue (TIS) should be monitored. The TIS assumes that only soft tissue is insonated. At 10 weeks after the last menstrual period, ossification of the fetal spine starts and the TIB should be monitored.
   b. **False.** Scanning with a TI between 0.7 and 1.0 is restricted to 60 min. There are no time restrictions for a TI <0.7.
   c. **True.**
   d. **False.** Scanning of the central nervous system (transcranial or spinal ultrasound) is not recommended with a TI >3.0. In this case, the thermal index for cranial imaging

(TIC) should be monitored. General neonatal scanning is not recommended with a TI >6.0. Note that, although allowed, scanning with a TI just below these values is unlikely to be of clinical use due to the time restrictions (e.g. general scanning with a TI between 4 and 5 is allowed for 15 s, and with a TI between 5 and 6 for 5 s only).

e. **False.** This possibility exists with an MI >0.3.

30. a. **True.** Note that the thermal index for soft tissue (TIS) should be monitored.
   b. **True.**
   c. **True.** Note that these values are the same as for neonatal ultrasound. The thermal index for cranial imaging (TIC) and thermal index for bone (TIB) should be used for central nervous system and general scanning, respectively.
   d. **False.** Consent is required of all patients, with verbal consent being generally acceptable. The British Medical Ultrasound Society recommends that, in the case of healthy volunteers, consent should ideally be expressed in a written form.
   e. **False.** The time should not exceed double that needed for a diagnostic examination.

Chapter

10

Magnetic resonance imaging – Questions

T. Matys and M. J. Graves

1. Regarding nuclear magnetic resonance imaging (MRI):
   a. In an external magnetic field, more hydrogen nuclei align with their magnetic moments parallel to the external field than antiparallel
   b. Protons subject to a strong static external magnetic field start to precess in phase
   c. The frequency of precession (Larmor frequency) of protons in a static magnetic field of 1.5 T equals 42.6 MHz
   d. At 1.5 T, the precessional frequency of hydrogen nuclei in fat is 220 Hz lower than that of hydrogen nuclei in water
   e. Apart from hydrogen, other nuclei that can be polarized in an external magnetic field include carbon ^{12}C and oxygen ^{16}O

2. Which of the following are true about MRI signal formation in biological tissues?
   a. A free induction decay (FID) signal can only occur after a 90° pulse
   b. After a 90° pulse, the longitudinal magnetization recovers at the same rate as the transverse magnetization decays
   c. The rate of the longitudinal magnetization recovery does not depend on the external magnetic field strength
   d. Dephasing of the transverse magnetization is mainly due to spin–lattice relaxation
   e. The FID is not usually considered in clinical MRI

3. In spin–echo (SE) imaging:
   a. The first radiofrequency pulse in a spin–echo pulse sequence is a 180° pulse
   b. Rephasing of the transverse magnetization is caused by the 180° pulse
   c. Effects of local field inhomogeneities on the MRI signal are eliminated
   d. For practical purposes, the delay between excitation and the refocusing pulse is kept constant, but signal readout can be performed at any chosen echo time (TE)
   e. Rephasing can only be performed once, and the whole sequence must be repeated to obtain another echo

4. Concerning image contrast in spin–echo imaging:
   a. The best contrast between tissues with different T_1s is obtained with short repetition times (TRs) and short echo times (TEs)
   b. T_2 weighting is obtained with short TEs and long TRs
   c. An image obtained with a TE of 15 ms and a TR of 2000 ms would be proton density (PD) weighted
   d. Fat appears with a high signal on T_1-, T_2- and PD-weighted sequences
   e. The fat signal is partially suppressed on fast (turbo) spin–echo imaging

5. Regarding relaxation times and the signal of different tissues:
   a. Cortical bone has long T_1 and T_2 relaxation times
   b. Water is hyperintense on both T_1- and T_2-weighted sequences
   c. Grey matter has a lower signal than white matter on T_1 sequences
   d. Melanoma metastases are usually of low T_2 signal
   e. Hyperacute intracerebral haemorrhage is bright on both T_1 and T_2 images

6. Regarding spatial encoding in standard (i.e. non-fast/turbo) spin–echo imaging:
   a. The slice-selection gradient is usually applied just before the 90° and 180° radiofrequency (RF) pulses
   b. A phase-encoding gradient is usually applied along the larger dimension of the imaged object
   c. The entire phase-encoded information is obtained during a single readout
   d. A frequency-encoding gradient is applied together with the phase-encoding gradient
   e. A spin–echo sequence requires a rephasing gradient applied after the slice-selection gradient

7. Concerning k-space:
   a. A line of data in k-space contains information corresponding to a particular phase-encoding step
   b. The central part of k-space contains information about low spatial frequencies
   c. Elimination of the periphery of the k-space would result in poor contrast but a sharp image
   d. One abnormally bright pixel in k-space would transform into a series of bright and dark circles originating from the centre of the final image
   e. The entire k-space must be acquired in order for the information to be transformed into a usable image

8. Regarding fast spin–echo (FSE)/turbo spin–echo (TSE) techniques:
   a. A fast spin–echo sequence involves a quick succession of multiple 90° pulses, each followed by a single refocusing pulse
   b. Rewinder gradients are used on the phase-encoding axis after each echo acquisition
   c. Contrast in the image can be affected by altering the order of k-space filling
   d. One of the most common applications of single-shot FSE techniques is MRCP
   e. Due to the short imaging time, fast spin–echo sequences lead to low energy deposition in tissues

9. Which of the following are true about gradient-recalled echo (GRE) in comparison with spin–echo sequences:
   a. Excitation flip angles less than 90° are generally used
   b. Imaging can be performed faster due to shorter TR times
   c. Rephasing of the spins and hence echo formation is achieved by using a phase-encoding gradient instead of a 180° pulse
   d. The excitation flip angle that maximizes the contrast between two tissues is known as the Ernst angle
   e. GRE is more prone to magnetic susceptibility artefacts than spin–echo sequences

10. Regarding types of gradient-recalled echo (GRE) sequence:
    a. Spoiled (incoherent) sequences allow T_1 weighting
    b. Spoiling can be achieved by pseudo-random variations in the phases of the excitation pulse
    c. Rewound (coherent) GRE sequences are useful in arthrographic, myelographic and angiographic applications
    d. Coherent sequences are insensitive to motion and flow
    e. Ultrafast spoiled gradient-echo sequences require magnetization preparation

11. Regarding echo-planar imaging (EPI):
    a. It allows the acquisition of high-resolution images
    b. Image formation is achieved by a series of alternating polarity gradients in the frequency-encoding direction
    c. Phase encoding is achieved by using gradients of varying strength that are rewound after each echo
    d. Different weightings can be achieved
    e. It is prone to artefacts

12. Which of the following are true regarding opposed-phase imaging?
    a. It is most commonly used with gradient-echo sequences
    b. In a 1.5 T magnet, the magnetization of fat and water becomes out of phase every 220 ms
    c. A gradient echo obtained with a TE of 6.9 ms at 1.5 T would represent a summation of signals from fat and water
    d. The most common application of out-of-phase imaging is in the diagnosis of hepatic and adrenal lesions
    e. Out-of-phase images show a characteristic 'India ink' appearance

13. Concerning inversion recovery:
    a. It can be used to achieve T_1 weighting or to suppress the signal from a specific tissue type
    b. The inversion recovery sequence starts with a 90° excitation pulse
    c. In short-TI inversion recovery (STIR) imaging, the TI is set equal to the T_1 of fat so that the signal from fat is nulled
    d. Image acquisition in FLAIR is usually combined with a T_2-weighted spin–echo sequence
    e. Inversion recovery sequences require high field magnets and are sensitive to magnetic field inhomogeneities

14. Regarding methods of fat suppression:
    a. The main advantage of short-TI inversion recovery (STIR) as a method of fat suppression is its specificity
    b. Out-of-phase imaging alone is useful for suppressing signal from adipose tissue
    c. Frequency-selective fat saturation is achieved by applying a chemical shift-selective excitation pulse followed by a spoiler gradient
    d. Higher magnetic field strengths allow better spectral fat saturation
    e. The signal-to-noise ratio (SNR) in images obtained with spectral fat saturation is worse in comparison with STIR

15. Regarding artefacts in MRI:
    a. Motion artefacts occur mainly in the frequency-encoding direction
    b. Aliasing usually occurs in the phase-encoding direction of 2D images
    c. Magnetic susceptibility effects are more pronounced on spin–echo than on gradient-echo sequences
    d. Chemical-shift artefacts are virtually eliminated in 3 T scanners
    e. Ringing (Gibbs) artefacts can be eliminated by increasing the matrix size

16. Signal-to-noise ratio (SNR) in MRI can be improved by:
    a. Increasing the tip angle in gradient-echo sequences above the Ernst angle
    b. Increasing the receiver bandwidth
    c. Using surface coils
    d. Using spin–echo sequences instead of gradient-recalled echo (GRE)
    e. Increasing the echo time (TE)

17. Which of the following are true regarding MRI parameters?
    a. Increasing voxel size increases signal-to-noise ratio (SNR)
    b. Decreasing the receiver bandwidth helps reduce chemical-shift artefacts
    c. The degree of improvement in the SNR is directly proportional to the number of repetitions
    d. Increasing the field strength improves the SNR
    e. Image contrast is dependent only on the T_1 and T_2 values of tissues

18. Regarding diffusion-weighted MRI (DW-MRI):
    a. Diffusion weighting is achieved by applying a single gradient pulse on the phase-encoding axis
    b. Areas of restricted diffusion show as a high signal on DW-MRI
    c. Interpretation of DW-MRI can be confounded by a 'shine-through' artefact
    d. Areas of restricted diffusion show as a high signal on an ADC map
    e. A pyogenic brain abscess has a high signal on DW-MRI

19. Regarding flow phenomena in MRI:
    a. Washout of blood from the imaged slice causes signal loss in both T_1-weighted spin–echo and gradient-echo imaging
    b. Fresh blood flowing into the slice causes flow enhancement on T_1-weighted gradient-echo sequences
    c. A bright intraluminal signal on T_1-weighted gradient-echo imaging confirms the vessel is patent
    d. Spin–echo imaging is better suited to assessment of the vessel wall than gradient-echo imaging
    e. Pulsatile flow is seen as ghosting artefacts in the phase-encoding direction

20. Which of the following are true about MRI contrast agents?
    a. Chelates of gadolinium are used in MRI due to their diamagnetic properties
    b. The mechanism of action of gadolinium involves shortening of the T_1 relaxation time
    c. Gadolinium-based contrast agents are eliminated mainly through renal excretion

   d. Iron oxide particles are used as negative-contrast agents

   e. Superparamagnetic iron oxide (SPIO) particles are used in contrast-enhanced angiography

21. Regarding nephrogenic systemic fibrosis (NSF):
   a. It usually involves the trunk first and spreads distally to the extremities
   b. It can occur in patients with normal kidney function
   c. The highest risk is posed by gadolinium compounds with a cyclical structure
   d. Most of the described cases are attributed to gadodiamide and gadopentetic acid
   e. In patients with severe renal impairment (estimated glomerular filtration rate (eGFR) <30 ml min^{-1} per 1.73 m^2), all gadolinium-based contrast agents are contraindicated

22. Concerning magnetic resonance angiography (MRA):
   a. Time-of-flight MRA (TOF-MRA) is used with gradient-echo sequences
   b. TOF-MRA is not prone to slow flow signal saturation
   c. Phase-contrast angiography (PCA) involves phase encoding by a monopolar gradient
   d. PCA allows imaging of slow-flowing blood
   e. Contrast-enhanced angiography is performed using fast gradient-echo sequences

23. In relation to specialized MRI techniques:
   a. Perfusion brain imaging is based on the differences between the magnetic properties of oxy- and deoxyhaemoglobin
   b. Brain perfusion imaging and functional imaging are usually performed with fast T_1-weighted sequences
   c. Areas of increased brain activity in functional BOLD imaging demonstrate a reduction in magnetic resonance (MR) signal
   d. MR spectroscopy requires a strong magnet that provides a uniform magnetic field
   e. MR spectroscopic images of ^{1}H, ^{31}P and ^{13}C can easily be obtained *in vivo*

24. Regarding permanent and resistive magnets:
   a. Permanent magnets used in MRI are often manufactured from ferrite
   b. Resistive magnets usually contain an iron yolk
   c. Typical strengths of the produced magnetic field are 0.2–0.3 T for permanent magnets and up to 1 T for resistive magnets
   d. At similar field strengths, the fringe field is more extensive in permanent than in resistive magnets
   e. The main use of permanent and resistive magnets is in open MRI systems

25. Concerning superconducting magnets:
   a. The coils of a superconducting magnet are usually made of niobium titanium (NbTi) in a copper matrix
   b. They are cooled by liquid nitrogen

   c. Once the magnetic field is established, no external electrical power is needed to maintain the current in the coils

   d. Modern designs use passive shielding to limit the extent of the fringe field

   e. A typical 1.5 T superconducting magnet provides a magnetic field that is 300,000 times stronger than that of the earth

26. Regarding types of coils used in MRI machines:
   a. Shim coils are used to actively shield the fringe field
   b. The typical noise emitted by a working MRI scanner is produced by the radiofrequency coils
   c. The body coil is always used as a transmitter coil
   d. Phased-array receiver coils allow a better signal-to-noise ratio (SNR) for a large field of view
   e. Phased-array surface coils allow parallel imaging

27. According to the UK Medicine and Healthcare products Regulatory Agency (MHRA) *Safety Guidelines for Magnetic Resonance Imaging Equipment in Clinical Use* (2007):
   a. The magnetic resonance (MR) controlled area contains the 0.5 mT (5 Gauss) field contour
   b. The inner MR controlled area contains the 5 mT (50 Gauss) field contour
   c. Ferromagnetic objects are allowed in the MR controlled area
   d. Persons with pacemakers can access the MR controlled area but not the inner MR controlled area
   e. Only equipment marked as 'MR Safe' can be brought into the inner MR controlled area

28. Regarding MRI risks and safety:
   a. The most often encountered adverse incidents in patients undergoing MR scanning in England are burns
   b. The main risk of the static magnetic field is its potential to cause a biological effect
   c. At field strengths of 3 T and higher, there is a potential risk for the function of artificial heart valves to be impaired due to the Lenz effect
   d. Peripheral nerve stimulation can occur in response to the radiofrequency fields
   e. The maximum allowed rise in total body temperature in the normal scanning mode is 0.5°C

29. Regarding the specific absorption ratio (SAR):
   a. The SAR defines the amount of energy deposited per kilogram of tissue by the time-varying magnetic field gradients
   b. The maximum allowed rise in body temperature in normal scanning is unlikely to be exceeded with an SAR <1 W kg^{-1}
   c. The SAR is higher in spin–echo imaging in comparison with gradient-recalled echo imaging
   d. The SAR can be reduced by using parallel imaging
   e. The SAR increases with repetition time (TR)

30. According to the UK Medicine and Healthcare products Regulatory Agency (MHRA) *Safety Guidelines for Magnetic Resonance Imaging Equipment in Clinical Use* (2007), an MRI examination is not allowed under any circumstances when the following is present:
    a. A pacemaker
    b. A hip/knee joint replacement
    c. An intracranial aneurysm clip
    d. A metallic heart valve
    e. A first-trimester pregnancy.

1. a. **True.** Slightly more hydrogen nuclei align parallel ('spin up') than antiparallel ('spin down'), giving rise to the net longitudinal magnetization M_Z. The difference between protons with parallel and antiparallel alignment is only 3 per million in a 1 T static magnetic field. This can be increased using special techniques (hyperpolarization).

   b. **False.** Protons align with the external field, but precess with different phases, cancelling each other's transverse magnetization. Therefore, the resulting net transverse magnetization (M_{XY}) is zero. Their phases are synchronized ('phase coherence') by an external 90° radiofrequency pulse whose frequency is equal to the Larmor frequency.

   c. **False.** This is the precessional frequency in a 1 T magnetic field. At 1.5 T, it would be proportionally higher, i.e. 63.9 MHz.

   d. **True.** This is called chemical shift and is utilized in some fat saturation techniques and opposed-phase imaging.

   e. **False.** Nuclear magnetic resonance is a property of nuclei with odd numbers of protons and/or neutrons (e.g. ^{13}C). Nuclei with even numbers of protons and neutrons have a zero net magnetic moment and cannot be polarized.

2. a. **False.** An FID will occur after any flip angle that results in a component of magnetization in the transverse plane. Only a 180° inversion pulse will not result in an FID.

   b. **False.** These two processes occur with different time constants termed T_1 and T_2, respectively, with T_2 being five to ten times shorter than T_1 in biological tissues.

   c. **False.** The stronger the external magnetic field, the longer the T_1 relaxation times.

   d. **False.** Dephasing occurs due to spin–spin interactions (T_2) and local magnetic field inhomogeneities. Spin–lattice (or T_1) relaxation is responsible for realignment of magnetic dipoles with the external magnetic field.

   e. **False.** Gradient-echo imaging involves sampling the signal formed during the FID. This is why gradient-echo images have a T_2^* weighting.

3. a. **False.** The first pulse is 90°, which tips the longitudinal magnetization into the transverse plane.

   b. **True.** The 180° pulse reverses the direction of spins. The spins gradually rephase resulting in 'regrowth' of the transverse magnetization vector M_{XY} and echo formation.

   c. **True.** This is because the 180° pulse reverses the dephasing due to field inhomogeneities.

    d. **False.** The TE is always double the time between the initial 90° and the 180° refocusing pulse. In order to obtain signals at different TEs, the timing between the radiofrequency pulses must be changed accordingly.

    e. **False.** Multiple refocusing 180° pulses can be applied following one excitation, and multiple echoes (albeit of decreasing amplitude due to T_2 relaxation) can be obtained. This is the basis of fast (turbo) spin–echo sequences.

4. a. **True.** T_1 weighting is obtained with a short TR, usually between 300 and 800 ms (close to the T_1s of the tissues being imaged). With increasing TR, the longitudinal magnetization in all tissues would recover more, diminishing the T_1 contrast. Short TEs are used to reduce the effect of T_2 relaxation on contrast (see below).

    b. **False.** Relatively long TEs (90–140 ms, close to the T_2s of the tissues being imaged) are used so measurable differences in the degree of transverse magnetization can develop. With short TEs, these differences are small; therefore, short TEs reduce the effect of T_2 weighing. Long TRs are used to allow near-full recovery of longitudinal magnetization and eliminate differences in contrast due to T_1.

    c. **True.** As described above, a short TE and long TR reduce the effect of T_2 and T_1, respectively. The remaining contrast is only dependent on the density of hydrogen nuclei (PD weighted).

    d. **True.** Due to a short T_1 and a higher PD in comparison with most tissues, fat is bright on these sequences. In T_2-weighted images, fat is less bright than water, but still brighter than most other tissues.

    e. **False.** On fast spin–echo images, fat appears hyperintense. This results from the multiple refocusing pulses, which suppress a phenomenon known as J-coupling (an interaction between different nuclei within the fat molecules), resulting in fat having a longer T_2 and therefore appearing brighter.

5. a. **False.** Cortical bone is essentially a solid, despite a water content of 10–15%. It has an extremely short T_2 of <1 ms; therefore, it appears black on conventional T_1- and T_2-weighted sequences.

    b. **False.** Water has a long T_1 and T_2; therefore, it appears hypointense on T_1 and hyperintense on T_2 sequences. This makes T_2 sequences sensitive for pathology, as most pathological processes (e.g. oedema, tumour, infarction) are associated with increased tissue water content.

    c. **True.** Grey matter has slightly longer T_1 and T_2 relaxation times than white matter, and so is darker on T_1 and brighter on T_2 sequences. The way to remember this is that grey matter is 'grey' on the sequence that better shows anatomy (T_1-weighted).

    d. **True.** There are only a few causes of a low T_2 signal; these include melanin, calcification, fibrous tissue, high protein content and flow void.

    e. **False.** The appearance of haemorrhage on T_1- and T_2-weighted imaging changes with time due to the temporal degradation of blood products according to the table on p. 135. Hyperacute blood is isointense or dark on T_1 and bright on T_2 sequence.

6. a. **False.** The slice selection gradient needs to be applied simultaneously and for the same duration as the RF pulses.

    b. **False.** If possible, phase encoding should be applied along the shorter dimension of the imaged object (i.e. lateral in head imaging, antero-posterior in abdominal

Temporal changes in the appearance of haemorrhage on MRI.

Timing	Blood product	T_1 signal	T_2 signal
Hyperacute	Oxyhaemoglobin	Isointense/hypointense	Hyperintense
Acute	Deoxyhaemoglobin	Isointense	Hypointense
Early subacute	Methaemoglobin (intracellular)	Hyperintense	Hypointense
Late subacute	Methaemoglobin (extracellular)	Hyperintense	Hyperintense
Chronic	Haemosiderin	Hypointense	Hypointense

imaging). This potentially allows a smaller number of phase-encoding steps (reduced-phase field of view) and minimizes the risk of aliasing artefacts.

c. **False.** Phase-encoded information is obtained in steps over the whole image acquisition.
d. **False.** It is applied during echo readout, while phase encoding is performed prior to it.
e. **True.** This is because the slice-selection gradient causes a phase shift along its direction arising during the second half of the gradient (after the magnetization is tipped into the transverse plane by the 90° pulse). This phase shift needs to be undone by an additional rephasing gradient with a reversed polarity and at half the area of the slice-selection gradient.

7. a. **True.**
   b. **True.** This contributes to the bulk of the image contrast.
   c. **False.** This would result in blurry images, i.e. poor spatial resolution, but contrast would be preserved. As contrast is more important for the final image, acquisition of the k-space periphery can sometimes be omitted to gain imaging speed, but sacrificing sharpness.
   d. **False.** This would transform into a sinusoidal signal modulation seen as parallel dark and bright lines with a periodicity dependent on the distance of the abnormal pixel from the k-space centre (the further from the centre, the higher the spatial frequency of the lines). This is often termed a 'herringbone' or 'corduroy' artefact, and may, for example, result from high-intensity radiofrequency spike noise originating from within the MRI room.
   e. **False.** It is sufficient to acquire just over one-half of the k-space. The missing part may be filled with zeros – this is known as zero filling and results in a blurry image. Alternatively, as k-space is symmetrical, the acquired half may be 'mirrored' (with appropriate mathematical corrections) into the missing half and the image reconstructed without loss of spatial resolution but with a decreased signal-to-noise ratio. This is sometimes known as half or fractional NEX (number of excitations) imaging.

8. a. **False.** It contains a single 90° excitation pulse followed by multiple refocusing pulses causing the formation of multiple echoes. The number of successive echoes (the echo train length or ETL) in extreme cases may equal the number of required phase-encoding steps, allowing acquisition of the entire image after a single 90° pulse (single-shot FSE). Acquisition can be accelerated further by using partial k-space filling (e.g. half-Fourier single-shot turbo spin–echo or HASTE).

b. **True.** The effect of the previous phase encoding needs to be reversed using a 'rewinder' gradient of equal but opposite area before the next refocusing pulse is applied.

c. **True.** Each echo in the train is acquired at increasing times from the 90° excitation pulse. The amplitude of each phase-encoding gradient is chosen such that the echoes nearest in time to the desired user-selected 'effective echo time (TE)' are placed in the centre of k-space (with the lowest amplitude of the phase-encoding gradient). The image contrast is therefore weighted to this 'effective TE'. Assuming a long repetition time (TR), if the centre of k-space is filled with the early echoes, then the effective TE is short and the image is proton density (PD) weighted. If the centre is filled with later echoes, then the effective TE is long and the images are T_2 weighted.

d. **True.** In single-shot FSE sequences, all the k-space data are acquired from a single 90° excitation pulse and a long train of refocusing pulses. If the echoes at the end of the train are used to fill the centre of the k-space, then the images become heavily T_2 weighted. In the abdomen, only tissues with long T_2 relaxation times will remain visible, i.e. fluid-filled structures such as the bile ducts, as the signal from other tissues will have decayed away. Other applications include uro-MRI and small-bowel MRI.

e. **False.** Due to the large number of refocusing pulses in a given TR, these sequences deposit substantial amounts of radiofrequency energy.

9. a. **True.** This allows shorter repetition times (TRs) to be used as not all the longitudinal magnetization is tipped into the transverse plane with each excitation. The image contrast is therefore dependent not only on echo time (TE) and TR but also on the flip angle.

b. **True.**

c. **False.** The echo is formed by a reversal of the frequency-encoding gradient. A prephasing gradient is used initially to dephase the spins, followed by the standard frequency-encoding gradient of the opposite polarity, which rephases the spins. Rephasing (and therefore signal amplitude) is maximal in the middle of the frequency-encoding gradient.

d. **False.** The Ernst angle is the excitation flip angle that maximizes the magnetic resonance signal for a given tissue T_1 and for a given TR. The Ernst angle (α_E) is given by $\cos(\alpha_E) = \exp(-TR/T_1)$. This angle may not necessarily provide the optimum contrast between any two tissues.

e. **True.** This is because local field inhomogeneities are not eliminated due to the absence of a 180° refocusing pulse.

10. a. **True.** If the repetition time (TR) is shorter than the T_2^* of the tissue, residual transverse magnetization remains at the time of the next radiofrequency (RF) excitation pulse. Spoiling eliminates this residual transverse magnetization and the image weighting becomes more T_1-like with increasing flip angle.

b. **True.** RF spoiling is the most common method for destroying transverse magnetization. Spoiling using various gradient 'killer' pulse schemes has been tried, but is not as effective. Examples of RF-spoiled sequences are SPGR (spoiled gradient recalled), FLASH (fast low-angle shot) and T_1-FFE (fast field echo).

c. **True.** These sequences preserve residual magnetization (steady state) by using a short TR and rewinding the phase-encoding gradient after the echo has been acquired so that there is no residual phase shift dependent on the phase-encoding step. The resulting signal is proportional to the ratio of T_2/T_1; therefore, water is hyperintense on these sequences, making them perfectly suited to these types of imaging. Other uses include 3D and breath-hold imaging. Examples of such sequences are GRE, FISP (fast imaging with steady-state precession) and FFE.

d. **False.** Motion and flow destroy the steady state on which these sequences depend.

e. **True.** Due to the very short TRs, in order not to saturate the transverse magnetization, only very small excitation flip angles are used, resulting in poor T_1 contrast. This can be overcome by applying preparation pulses, such as a 180° inversion prior to acquisition, which improves the T_1 contrast between tissues.

11. a. **False.** An acquisition matrix resolution is usually limited to 64 × 64 or 128 × 128.

b. **True.** The polarity of the frequency-encoding gradient is repeatedly changed so that the k-space is traversed in a backwards–forwards (raster) fashion.

c. **False.** A small but constant phase-encoding gradient is applied after each echo formation to move the k-space trajectory up one step. This is often referred to as a 'blip'.

d. **True.** EPI can be weighted for T_2, T_2^*, T_1 or diffusion.

e. **True.** It is particularly prone to chemical shift artefacts that need to be prevented by fat suppression and to artefacts resulting from non-perfect alignment of the forward and reverse echoes ('N/2 ghosting').

12. a. **True.** It relies on the phase differences arising due to different resonance frequencies of water and fat. The echo time (TE) is chosen such that the echo forms when the water and fat signals have a 180° phase difference between them. In standard spin–echo sequences, these phase differences would be eliminated by the 180° refocusing pulse.

b. **False.** The difference in Larmor frequency between fat and water at 1.5 T is approximately 220 Hz. Fat and water will therefore be in phase at every multiple of $1000/220 = 4.6$ ms (i.e. at 4.6, 9.2, 13.8 ms, etc.). Hence, they will be out of phase mid-way between these time points (i.e. at 2.3, 6.9, 11.5 ms etc.).

c. **False.** At this time point, fat and water are out of phase, so the resulting signal would represent the difference in the fat and water magnetizations in that voxel.

d. **True.** Fatty lesions of these organs that contain both fat and water will show signal hypointensity on the out-of-phase images in comparison with the corresponding in-phase images.

e. **True.** At interfaces where voxels contain both water and fat, in the out-of-phase images the magnetization cancels, resulting in a one-voxel thin black line as if drawn with ink.

13. a. **True.** Inversion recovery with a TI (inversion time, originally called tau time) of around 500 ms can be used as magnetization preparation for T_1 weighting, for example before a turbo gradient-echo sequence. By varying the TI, it may also be used to suppress the signal from a specific tissue, most commonly from fat (in short-TI inversion recovery or STIR imaging) or cerebrospinal fluid (in fluid attenuation inversion recovery or FLAIR).

b. **False.** It starts with inversion of the longitudinal magnetization (M_Z) by a 180° radiofrequency (RF) pulse.

c. **False.** following the 180° inversion pulse, the magnetization relaxes due to T_1 recovery and crosses zero at a time equal to $0.693 \times T_1$ of the given tissue. Applying the excitation pulse at this particular time results in no signal from the specific tissue as there is no net magnetization to be flipped into the transverse plane. As the T_1 of fat is approximately 220 ms at 1.5 T, using an inversion recovery sequence with a TI of $0.693 \times 220 \approx 150$ ms results in zero signal from fat.

d. **True.** FLAIR suppresses the high signal from cerebrospinal fluid in T_2-weighted imaging resulting in increased conspicuity of demyelinating periventricular brain lesions.

e. **False.** They work well with low field strength magnets and are not sensitive to static magnetic field inhomogeneities as they work on the basis of differences in T_1 relaxation times.

14. a. **False.** STIR is not specific and the signal from all tissues with a T_1 close to that of fat will be suppressed; these include mucoid tissue, haemorrhage, protein-rich fluid and gadolinium or melanin at specific concentrations.

b. **False.** On its own, out-of-phase imaging is only useful in suppressing signals from voxels containing a mixture of fat and water, mainly for diagnostic purposes.

c. **True.** This selectively tips the longitudinal magnetization of fat into the transverse plane, where it is dephased by a spoiler gradient before the excitation pulse is applied. Fat therefore cannot contribute to the signal in the image.

d. **True.** The chemical shift between fat and water is proportional to field strength; therefore, the use of a higher magnetic field strength makes the design of frequency-selective pulses easier and avoids the risk of unwanted saturation of the water signal. This is why chemical shift-selective saturation pulses are not normally used at lower field strengths, e.g. less than approximately 0.3 T.

e. **False.** The signal from non-adipose tissue is virtually unaffected by frequency-selective fat saturation. In contrast, an inversion recovery pulse affects magnetization of all tissues, lowering the overall SNR.

15. a. **False.** Motion artefacts occur in the phase-encoding direction regardless of the actual direction of motion and are usually seen as either a smearing (induced by random motion) or ghosting (periodic motion).

b. **True.** Aliasing is encountered in the phase-encoding direction when a part of the patient that lies beyond the chosen field of view appears on the opposite side of the image (known as a wrap-around artefact). A field of view smaller than the object in the frequency-encoding direction does not exhibit aliasing as the frequency-encoded signals are electronically filtered to remove the frequencies outside the receiver bandwidth. Note that in 3D scans, aliasing can also occur in the slice-select direction, as 3D slice encoding also relies on a phase shift.

c. **False.** Magnetic susceptibility artefacts are worse on gradient-echo sequences, which do not provide compensation for local magnetic field inhomogeneities.

d. **False.** Because the chemical shift (difference in resonance frequency) between fat and water is proportional to the static magnetic field strength, the resulting artefacts may be more pronounced at higher field strengths.

e. **True.** Ringing appears as alternating dark and bright lines parallel to a high-contrast interface and is due to insufficient sampling of higher spatial frequencies. It can occur along the frequency- or phase-encoding direction, but is more commonly seen in the latter (due to the phase matrix being smaller in order to reduce scanning time).

16. a. **False.** The Ernst angle is the flip angle at which the signal is maximal for a given T_1 and repetition time (TR). Increasing the flip angle above this value would lead to a decrease in signal.
  b. **False.** SNR is inversely proportional to the square root of the bandwidth. A larger bandwidth increases the detected noise.
  c. **True.** This reduces the volume of tissue from which noise is detected.
  d. **True.** In general, spin echo gives higher signal than GRE.
  e. **False.** As the TE increases, more T_2 decay occurs resulting in a smaller signal.

17. a. **True.** The signal will increase at the expense of a reduction in spatial resolution.
  b. **False.** Decreasing the receiver bandwidth decreases the strength of the frequency-encoding gradient resulting in a larger chemical shift between water and fat.
  c. **False.** It is proportional to the square root of the number of repetitions. Thus, repeating the sequence four times would result in a twofold improvement in the SNR.
  d. **True.** As a first approximation, the SNR increases linearly with magnetic field strength.
  e. **False.** There are a number of methods to improve image contrast, including fat suppression, magnetization transfer and the use of contrast media. Image contrast will also depend on the chosen echo and repetition times, which will determine the image weighting.

18. a. **False.** Diffusion weighting is achieved by applying a pair of diffusion-encoding gradients on either side of the 180° pulse in a spin–echo echo-planar imaging (EPI) sequence. It is generally necessary to apply the diffusion gradients separately on all three orthogonal axes in order to eliminate effects due to diffusion anisotropy.
  b. **True.** The effect of the diffusion gradients is to reduce the overall image intensity due to irreversible signal loss caused by spins diffusing in the presence of the two diffusion gradients. In regions of restricted diffusion, such as cytotoxic oedema secondary to a stroke, the distance the spins can diffuse is reduced and hence the signal loss is not as great, resulting in regions of relative hyperintensity compared with normal tissue.
  c. **True.** The requirement for the large (high amplitude and long duration) diffusion gradients increases the effective echo time (TE) making the DW-MRI T_2 weighted. Therefore the high signal of water may sometimes be misinterpreted as restricted diffusion. Calculation of an apparent diffusion coefficient (ADC) map can eliminate the effect of this T_2 shine-through.
  d. **False.** Areas of restricted diffusion on an ADC map are hypointense. The ADC map is calculated from two diffusion sequences obtained with different *b*-values, and is independent of T_2.
  e. **True.** DW-MRI is therefore helpful in distinguishing a brain abscess (with a restricted diffusion) from a necrotic metastasis, which usually exhibits unrestricted diffusion.

19. a. **False.** Washout of blood from the slice between the 90° and 180° pulses in spin–echo imaging causes signal loss because the blood will not have experienced both the 90° and 180° pulses in order to produce a spin echo. In gradient-echo imaging, only one radiofrequency pulse is required for signal formation so there is no washout phenomenon.
   b. **True.** This is because the inflowing fresh blood has full longitudinal magnetization, which will produce a high signal compared with the stationary background tissue.
   c. **False.** Any tissue that has a short T_1 can appear bright on T_1-weighted gradient-echo imaging. It is therefore possible that blood breakdown products such as methaemoglobin could give a bright intraluminal signal that could be misinterpreted as blood flowing in a patent vessel.
   d. **True.** This is because fast-flowing blood appears dark due to flow washout (black blood imaging) allowing good visualization of the vessel wall.
   e. **True.** Ghosting artefacts produced by periodic motion occur along the phase-encoding axis.

20. a. **False.** Gadolinium ions are paramagnetic, which means that they have a large electron magnetic moment that can cause rapid T_1 relaxation in nearby protons.
   b. **True.** Therefore, they cause signal enhancement in regions of gadolinium accumulation on T_1-weighted sequences.
   c. **True.** Most are eliminated via the kidneys. Some agents (e.g. gadoxetic acid) are also excreted with bile.
   d. **True.** Iron oxide nanoparticles are superparamagnetic. They have been used as negative-contrast agents due to their strong susceptibility effect, which shortens T_2 and T_2^* relaxation time of nearby protons.
   e. **False.** SPIO particles are taken up by the reticulo-endothelial system of the liver (Kupfer cells) and are used in the diagnosis of hepatic tumours. Ultra-small SPIOs (USPIOs) accumulate mainly in lymph nodes, but their small size also makes them potentially useful as blood pool agents for magnetic resonance angiography (MRA). However, they are not currently commercially available for this application.

21. a. **False.** NSF starts as fibrosis of the skin and connective tissue of the extremities.
   b. **False.** There are no known cases of NSF in patients with normal kidney function.
   c. **False.** NSF is thought to be associated with the release of free Gd^{3+} from the chelate. This is most likely to happen with linear non-ionic compounds, and is least likely with cyclic compounds.
   d. **True.** Most cases have been associated with gadiodiamide (Omniscan). A small number of cases have been associated with gadopentetic acid (Magnevist).
   e. **False.** According to the guidance from the UK Medicine and Healthcare products Regulatory Agency (MHRA), such patients should not be given gadodiamide and gadopentetic acid. In the case of other gadolinium-containing compounds, 'careful consideration should be given'.

22. a. **True.** Due to the time-of-flight effect causing flow enhancement on these sequences, this provides a good signal from blood vessels. The signal from stationary tissue is saturated with large flip angles, which further improves contrast.
   b. **False.** Slow-flowing blood, especially parallel to the slice, may become saturated leading to loss of signal. This is one of the main limitations of TOF-MRA.

c. **False.** Bipolar gradients are used – these cause a phase shift in spins moving along the direction of the gradient without affecting stationary spins. Two acquisitions are obtained in each direction with reversed polarity of the bipolar gradient to eliminate field inhomogeneities.

d. **True.** Unlike TOF-MRA, PCA is not prone to saturation and slow-flowing blood can be imaged.

e. **True.**

23. a. **False.** This forms the basis of brain oxygenation level dependent (BOLD) functional imaging (see below). Perfusion imaging is based on a susceptibility effect (shortening of T_2^* time upon first passage of an exogenous contrast agent) or on arterial spin labelling (inversion of the longitudinal magnetization of blood upstream of the investigated organ).

b. **False.** Sequences sensitive to magnetic susceptibility, i.e. T_2^* weighting, are used.

c. **False.** The BOLD effect relies on different magnetic characteristics of oxyhaemoglobin (diamagnetic) and deoxyhaemoglobin (paramagnetic). When the metabolic activity of the brain increases, there is a slight increase in deoxyhaemoglobin production but a disproportionately larger increase in blood flow (due to neurovascular coupling) carrying oxyhaemoglobin. The net effect is an increase in MR signal on T_2^*-weighted sequences due to the increase in diamagnetic oxyhaemoglobin over the resting-state level of paramagnetic deoxyhaemoglobin.

d. **True.** It is based on measuring chemical shift (changes in resonance frequency of protons in different compounds), which is proportional to the strength of the external magnetic field. The field must be uniform to better than 1 ppm.

e. **False.** While ^1H and ^{31}P spectroscopy is possible, spectroscopic imaging of ^{13}C is impractical due to the low signal-to-noise ratio and natural abundance. In the future, imaging of ^{13}C may be possible using hyperpolarization techniques.

24. a. **False.** They are usually made from rare earth materials – typically neodymium-iron-boron (NIB) or samarium cobalt (SmCo).

b. **True.** Old air-cored designs are no longer in use.

c. **False.** The value for permanent magnets is correct; however, currently available iron-cored resistive magnets give field strengths of up to 0.6 T only.

d. **False.** In permanent magnets, the fringe field is almost entirely contained within the magnet.

e. **True.**

25. a. **True.** The superconducting NbTi wires are embedded in a copper matrix, which thermally protects them in the event of a quench (the case of a sudden loss of superconductivity).

b. **False.** They are cooled by liquid helium (boiling point 4.2 K). Liquid nitrogen (boiling point 77 K) does not provide a low enough temperature for the NbTi alloy to become superconductive. Liquid nitrogen was used in older designs of magnets to help reduce the boil-off of the more expensive helium.

c. **True.**

d. **False.** Modern designs are actively shielded by additional superconducting coils that are placed inside the magnet cryostat but have current flowing in the opposite direction so as to reduce the field outside the magnet.

e. **False.** The typical field strength (1.5 T) is 30,000 times stronger than that of the earth's magnetic field (typically 50 μT).

26. a. **False.** Their purpose is to improve the uniformity of the static magnetic field.
    b. **False.** This is owing to the gradient coils mechanically flexing (Lorentz force) due to currents being passed through them during imaging.
    c. **False.** Smaller transmitter coils are sometimes used for imaging of the head and limbs.
    d. **True.** Phased-array coils consist of a number of smaller coils that can be applied as a surface coil. The array allows a large field of view, with the higher SNR of the individual smaller coils.
    e. **True.** Parallel-imaging techniques use phased-array coils to decrease the number of phase-encoding steps; examples include image-based parallel reconstruction (SENSE) and k-space-based reconstruction (generalized autocalibrating partially parallel acquisition or GRAPPA).

27. a. **True.**
    b. **False.** This contains the 3 mT (30 Gauss) field contour.
    c. **True.** However, they cannot be brought into the inner MR controlled area where a projectile hazard exists. Good practice would indicate that ferromagnetic objects are also kept out of the controlled area.
    d. **False.** Patients with pacemakers are not allowed to be exposed to a magnetic field stronger than 0.5 mT (MR controlled area; note this can extend beyond the actual MR room). This may change in the future given the availability of MRI-compatible pacemakers.
    e. **False.** Equipment marked as 'MR Conditional' can also be brought into the inner controlled area, providing the specified conditions are met.

28. a. **True.** This is due to eddy currents arising in conducting loops. Burns can also occur where the arms and legs are touching, forming a conducting loop pathway.
    b. **False.** The main risk is that of a ferromagnetic object entering the inner MR controlled area becoming a projectile.
    c. **True.** The Lenz effect is an induction of a magnetic field in a moving conductor that opposes the external magnetic field. It is of low significance at a 1.5 T field, but is a potential hazard at higher field strengths.
    d. **False.** This is caused by magnetic field gradients.
    e. **True.** In the first-level controlled mode with appropriate monitoring, the allowable temperature rise is 1°C.

29. a. **False.** Energy is mainly deposited by the radiofrequency (RF) fields.
    b. **True.** For shorter exposure times (<15 min) the limit is < 2 W kg^{-1}.
    c. **True.** This is especially true in fast/turbo spin–echo imaging. Reducing the echo train length decreases the energy deposition.
    d. **True.** Parallel imaging can reduce RF exposure due to the decrease in the number of RF pulses used.
    e. **False.** Longer TRs reduce the duty cycle and allow time for the tissue to cool down.

30. a. **True**. According to the most recent MHRA guidance, patients with implanted pacemakers must not be examined by magnetic resonance (MR) diagnostic equipment. No provision is currently made for MR-safe pacemakers.
   b. **False**. Patients should be monitored carefully; heat generation in the prosthesis is a potential problem.
   c. **False**. Patients with non-ferromagnetic clips (titanium, tantalum, vanadium) can be examined.
   d. **False**. The force from the external magnetic field is minimal compared with the force exerted by the beating heart.
   e. **False**. The decision to scan should be based on the balance of clinical benefit and risks (which remain unknown, with excessive heating being potentially harmful).

Bibliography

General

Allisy-Roberts P, Williams J. *Farr's Physics for Medical Imaging*, 2nd edn. Edinburgh: Saunders, 2007.

Baert AL. *Encyclopedia of Diagnostic Imaging*. Berlin: Springer Verlag, 2007.

Bushberg JT. *The Essential Physics of Medical Imaging*. Philadelphia: Lippincott Williams & Wilkins, 2002.

Hendee WR, Ritenour ER. *Medical Imaging Physics*, 4th edn. New York: Wiley-Blackwell, 2002.

Radiology – Integrated Training Initiative (R-ITI). e-Learning for Healthcare: http://www.e-lfh.org.uk/projects/radiology/index.html.

Film-screen radiography/Digital radiography/Imaging with X-rays

Department of Health, April 2007. Guidance on the establishment and use of diagnostic reference levels: http://www.dh.gov.uk/en/Publicationsandstatistics/Publications/PublicationsPolicyAndGuidance/DH_074067

Kuhlman KE, Collins J, Brooks GN, Yandow DR, Broderick LS. Dual energy subtraction chest radiography: what to look for beyond calcified nodules. *Radiographics* 2006; **26**:79–92.

The Royal College of Radiologists IT guidance (June 2010)

- Radiology Information Systems: http://www.rcr.ac.uk/docs/radiology/pdf/IT_guidance_RISApr08.pdf
- Storage requirements and solutions for PACS: http://www.rcr.ac.uk/docs/radiology/pdf/ITguidance_Storage_Requirements_PACS.pdf
- PACS and quality assurance: http://www.rcr.ac.uk/docs/radiology/pdf/IT_guidance_QAApr08.pdf
- PACS and guidance on diagnostic display devices: http://www.rcr.ac.uk/docs/radiology/pdf/IT_guidance_PACSApr08.pdf

Ultrasound imaging

British Medical Ultrasound Society (BMUS). Safety Guidelines (2009): http://www.bmus.org/policies-guides/BMUS-Safety-Guidelines-2009-revision-FINAL-Nov-2009.pdf (accessed 16 June 2010).

Cosgrove D. Ultrasound contrast agents: an overview. *European Journal of Radiology* 2006; **60**:324–330.

Dähnert W. *Radiology Review Manual*, 6th edn. Philadelphia: Lippincott Williams & Wilkins, 2007.

European Federation of Societies for Ultrasound in Medicine and Biology. Guidelines and Good Clinical Practice Recommendations for Contrast Enhanced Ultrasound (CEUS): http://www.efsumb.org/mediafiles01/cues-guidelines2008.pdf (accessed 16 June 2010).

Hoskins PR, Martin K, Thrush A. *Diagnostic Ultrasound: Physics and Equipment*. Cambridge: Cambridge University Press, 2003.

Kollmann C. New sonographic techniques for harmonic imaging – underlying physical principles. European Journal of Radiology 2007; **64**:164–172.

Szabo T. *Diagnostic Ultrasound Imaging: Inside Out*. Burlington, MA: Elsevier Academic Press, 2004.

144

The Royal College of Radiologists. Standards for Ultrasound Equipment: http://www.rcr.ac.uk/docs/radiology/pdf/StandardsforUltrasoundEquipmentJan2005.pdf (accessed 16 June 2010).

Tran TD, Caruthers SD, Hughes M, Marsh JN, Cyrus T, Winter PM, Neubauer AM, Wickline SA Lanza GM. Clinical applications of perfluorocarbon nanoparticles for molecular imaging and targeted therapeutics. *International Journal of Nanomedicine* 2007; 2:515–526.

Magnetic resonance imaging

McRobbie DW, Moore EA, Graves MJ, Prince MR. *MRI from Picture to Proton*. Cambridge: Cambridge University Press, 2007.

Medicines and Healthcare products Regulatory Agency (MHRA). Nephrogenic Systemic Fibrosis (NSF) and gadolinium-containing MRI contrast agents: http://www.mhra.gov.uk/Safetyinformation/Safetywarningsalertsandrecalls/Safetywarningsandmessagesformedicines/CON2030229 (accessed 27 May 2010).

Medicines and Healthcare products Regulatory Agency (MHRA). Nephrogenic Systemic Fibrosis (NSF) with gadolinium-containing magnetic resonance imaging (MRI) contrast agents – Update: http://www.mhra.gov.uk/Safetyinformation/Safetywarningsalertsandrecalls/Safetywarningsandmessagesformedicines/CON2031543 (accessed 27 May 2010).

Medicines and Healthcare products Regulatory Agency (MHRA). DB 2007(03) Safety guidelines for magnetic resonance imaging equipment in clinical use: http://www.mhra.gov.uk/Publications/Safetyguidance/DeviceBulletins/CON2033018 (accessed 29 May 2010).

Index

Printed in the United States
by Baker & Taylor Publisher Services